Takotsubo Syndrome

Editors

EDUARDO BOSSONE
RAIMUND ERBEL

HEART FAILURE CLINICS

www.heartfailure.theclinics.com

Consulting Editors
MANDEEP R. MEHRA
JAVED BUTLER

Founding Editor
JAGAT NARULA

October 2016 • Volume 12 • Number 4

ELSEVIER

1600 John F. Kennedy Boulevard • Suite 1800 • Philadelphia, Pennsylvania, 19103-2899

http://www.theclinics.com

HEART FAILURE CLINICS Volume 12, Number 4
October 2016 ISSN 1551-7136, ISBN-13: 978-0-323-46312-6

Editor: Lauren Boyle
Developmental Editor: Alison Swety

Heart Failure Clinics (ISSN 1551-7136) is published quarterly by Elsevier Inc., 360 Park Avenue South, New York, NY 10010-1710. Months of publication are January, April, July, and October. Business and editorial offices: 1600 John F. Kennedy Boulevard, Suite 1800, Philadelphia, PA 19103-2899. Periodicals postage paid at New York, NY, and additional mailing offices. Subscription prices are USD 240.00 per year for US individuals, USD 431.00 per year for US institutions, USD 100.00 per year for US students and residents, USD 280.00 per year for Canadian individuals, USD 499.00 per year for Canadian institutions, USD 300.00 per year for international individuals, USD 499.00 per year for international institutions, and USD 100.00 per year for Canadian and foreign students/residents. To receive student and resident rate, orders must be accompanied by name of affiliated institution, date of term, and the *signature* of program/residency coordinator on institution letterhead. Orders will be billed at individual rate until proof of status is received. Foreign air speed delivery is included in all *Clinics* subscription prices. All prices are subject to change without notice. **POSTMASTER:** Send address changes to *Heart Failure Clinics*, Elsevier Health Sciences Division, Subscription Customer Service, 3251 Riverport Lane, Maryland Heights, MO 63043. **Customer Service: 1-800-654-2452 (US and Canada). From outside of the US and Canada, call 314-447-8871. Fax: 314-447-8029. For print support, E-mail: JournalsCustomerService-usa@elsevier.com. For online support, E-mail: JournalsOnlineSupport-usa@elsevier.com.**

Reprints. For copies of 100 or more of articles in this publication, please contact the Commercial Reprints Department, Elsevier Inc., 360 Park Avenue South, New York, NY 10010-1710. Tel.: 212-633-3874; Fax: 212-633-3820; E-mail: reprints@elsevier.com.

Heart Failure Clinics is covered in *MEDLINE/PubMed (Index Medicus)*.

Contributors

CONSULTING EDITORS

MANDEEP R. MEHRA, MD, FACC, FACP, FRCP
Heart and Vascular Center, Brigham and Women's Hospital, Harvard Medical School, Boston, Massachusetts

JAVED BUTLER, MD, MPH, MBA
Stony Brook University Heart Institute, Department of Internal Medicine, Stony Brook School of Medicine, Stony Brook University Medical Center, Stony Brook, New York

EDITORS

EDUARDO BOSSONE, MD, PhD, FCCP, FESC, FACC
Cardiology Division, "Cava de' Tirreni and Amalfi Coast," Heart Department, University Hospital, Cava de' Tirreni (SA), Italy

RAIMUND ERBEL, MD, FAHA, FESC, FACC, FASE
Institute of Medical Informatics Biometry and Epidemiology, University Clinic Essen, Essen, Germany

AUTHORS

YOSHIHIRO J. AKASHI, MD, PhD, FESC, FJCC
Professor, Division of Cardiology, Department of Internal Medicine, St. Marianna University School of Medicine, Kawasaki, Kanagawa, Japan

IBRAHIM AKIN, MD
First Department of Medicine, Medical Faculty Mannheim, University Heidelberg; DZHK (German Center for Cardiovascular Research), Partner Site, Heidelberg-Mannheim, Mannheim, Germany

SATPAL ARRI, MBBS, MRCP
Cardiovascular Division, Rayne Institute, King's College London, St Thomas' Hospital, London, United Kingdom

MARTIN BORGGREFE, MD
First Department of Medicine, Medical Faculty Mannheim, University Heidelberg; DZHK (German Center for Cardiovascular Research),

Partner Site, Heidelberg-Mannheim, Mannheim, Germany

EDUARDO BOSSONE, MD, PhD, FCCP, FESC, FACC
Cardiology Division, "Cava de' Tirreni and Amalfi Coast," Heart Department, University Hospital, Cava de' Tirreni (SA), Italy

PAOLO CALABRÒ, MD, PhD, FESC
Cardiologia SUN, Monaldi Hospital, AORN dei Colli, Second University of Naples, Naples, Italy

RAFFAELE CALABRÒ, MD
Cardiologia SUN, Monaldi Hospital, AORN dei Colli, Second University of Naples, Naples, Italy

VICTORIA L. CAMMANN
Department of Cardiology, University Heart Center, University Hospital Zurich, Zurich, Switzerland

ANNAPAOLA CIRILLO, MD
Cardiologia SUN, Monaldi Hospital, AORN dei Colli, Second University of Naples, Naples, Italy

RODOLFO CITRO, MD, PhD
Department of Cardiology, University Hospital "San Giovanni di Dio e Ruggi d'Aragona," Salerno, Italy

GUIDO RONALD COPPOLA, MD
Cardiologia SUN, Monaldi Hospital, AORN dei Colli, Second University of Naples, Naples, Italy

ABHISHEK J. DESHMUKH, MBBS
Assistant Professor of Medicine, Mayo Clinic Heart Rhythm Section, Cardiovascular Diseases, Mayo Clinic, Rochester, Minnesota

IBRAHIM EL-BATTRAWY, MD
First Department of Medicine, Medical Faculty Mannheim, University Heidelberg; DZHK (German Center for Cardiovascular Research), Partner Site, Heidelberg-Mannheim, Mannheim, Germany

FABIO FABBIAN, MD
Assistant Professor, Clinica Medica Unit, School of Medicine, University of Ferrara, Ferrara, Italy

FIORELLA FRATTA, MD
Cardiologia SUN, Monaldi Hospital, AORN dei Colli, Second University of Naples, Naples, Italy

ADELAIDE FUSCO, MD
Cardiologia SUN, Monaldi Hospital, AORN dei Colli, Second University of Naples, Naples, Italy

MASSIMO GALLERANI, MD
Chief, 1st Internal Unit of Internal Medicine, General Hospital of Ferrara, Ferrara, Italy

JELENA-R. GHADRI, MD
Department of Cardiology, University Heart Center, University Hospital Zurich, Zurich, Switzerland

MASAHARU ISHIHARA, MD, PhD, FACC, FJCC
Professor, Division of Coronary Artery Disease, Department of Internal Medicine, Hyogo College of Medicine, Nishinomiya, Hyogo, Japan

GIUSEPPE LIMONGELLI, MD, PhD, FESC
Cardiologia SUN, Monaldi Hospital, AORN dei Colli, Second University of Naples, Naples, Italy

SPINELLI BARRILE LUDOVICA, MD
Cardiologia SUN, Monaldi Hospital, AORN dei Colli, Second University of Naples, Naples, Italy

ALEXANDER R. LYON, MA, BM BCh, PhD, FRCP
Senior Lecturer and Consultant Cardiologist, National Institute for Health Research Cardiovascular Biomedical Research Unit, Royal Brompton & Harefield NHS Foundation Trust, National Heart & Lung Institute, Imperial College London, London, United Kingdom

VALERIA MADDALONI, MD
Genomic and Cellular Lab, Monaldi Hospital, AORN dei Colli, Second University of Naples, Naples, Italy

FABIO MANFREDINI, MD
Assistant Professor, Department of Biomedical Sciences and Surgical Specialties, Vascular Diseases Center, School of Medicine, University of Ferrara, Ferrara, Italy

ROBERTO MANFREDINI, MD
Full Professor of Internal Medicine and Chief, Clinica Medica Unit, School of Medicine, University of Ferrara, Ferrara, Italy

DANIELE MASARONE, MD
Cardiologia SUN, Monaldi Hospital, AORN dei Colli, Second University of Naples, Naples, Italy

ANDREW C. MORLEY-SMITH, MA, MB BChir, MRCP
Clinical Research Fellow, National Institute for Health Research Cardiovascular Biomedical Research Unit, Royal Brompton & Harefield NHS Foundation Trust, National Heart & Lung Institute, Imperial College London, London, United Kingdom

ELMIR OMEROVIC, MD, PhD
Department of Molecular and Clinical Medicine, Institute of Medicine, Sahlgrenska Academy, University of Gothenburg; Associate Professor of Cardiology, Department of Cardiology, Sahlgrenska University Hospital, Gothenburg, Sweden

LEONARDO PACE, MD
Department of Medicine and Surgery, Schola Medica Salernitana, University of Salerno, Salerno, Italy

GIUSEPPE PACILEO, MD
Cardiologia SUN, Monaldi Hospital, AORN dei Colli, Second University of Naples, Naples, Italy

ROBERTA PACILEO, MD
Cardiologia SUN, Monaldi Hospital, AORN dei Colli, Second University of Naples, Naples, Italy

FRANCESCA PISACANE, MD
Cardiologia SUN, Monaldi Hospital, AORN dei Colli, Second University of Naples, Naples, Italy

FEDERICO PISCIONE, MD
Department of Medicine and Surgery, Schola Medica Salernitana, University of Salerno; Department of Cardiology, University Hospital "San Giovanni di Dio e Ruggi d'Aragona," Salerno, Italy

GIANLUCA PONTONE, MD, PhD
Monzino Cardiac Centre, IRCCS, Milan, Italy

ABHIRAM PRASAD, MD, FRCP, FACC, FESC
Professor of Interventional Cardiology, Cardiovascular and Cell Sciences Research Institute, St. George's, University of London, London, United Kingdom

MARTA RUBINO, MD
Cardiologia SUN, Monaldi Hospital, AORN dei Colli, Second University of Naples, Naples, Italy

MARIA GIOVANNA RUSSO, MD
Cardiologia SUN, Monaldi Hospital, AORN dei Colli, Second University of Naples, Naples, Italy

RAFFAELLA SALMI, MD
Chief, 2nd Internal Unit of Internal Medicine, General Hospital of Ferrara, Ferrara, Italy

BIRKE SCHNEIDER, MD
Medizinische Klinik II, Sana Kliniken Lübeck, Lübeck, Germany

UDO SECHTEM, MD
Abteilung für Kardiologie, Robert-Bosch-Krankenhaus, Stuttgart, Germany

SCOTT W. SHARKEY, MD
Cardiovascular Research Division, Minneapolis Heart Institute Foundation, Minneapolis, Minnesota

ANGELO SILVERIO, MD
Department of Cardiology, University Hospital "San Giovanni di Dio e Ruggi d'Aragona," Salerno, Italy

CHRISTIAN TEMPLIN, MD, PhD
Department of Cardiology, University Heart Center, University Hospital Zurich, Zurich, Switzerland

RUPERT WILLIAMS, MBBS, MRCP, PhD
Cardiovascular and Cell Sciences Research Institute, St. George's, University of London, London, United Kingdom

ILAN S. WITTSTEIN, MD
Assistant Professor of Medicine, Division of Cardiology, The Johns Hopkins University School of Medicine, Baltimore, Maryland

CONCETTA ZITO, MD, PhD
Cardiology, Department of Clinical and Experimental Medicine, University of Messina, Messina, Italy

Contents

Rupert Williams, Satpal Arri, and Abhiram Prasad

Takotsubo syndrome is typically characterized by acute reversible impairment of apical and mid-left ventricular systolic function. The pathophysiology is complex and remains to be completely understood. A catecholamine surge appears to be a central feature. Patients with prior history of psychiatric disorders have a predisposition. The putative role of a switch in b-adrenoceptor signalling resulting in negative inotropy remains uncertain. Downregulation of noncritical cellular functions may offer some protection in preventing irreversible cellular necrosis. Microvascular function is a common occurrence in these patients.

Ilan S. Wittstein

Takotsubo syndrome is a unique clinical condition of acute heart failure and reversible left ventricular dysfunction frequently precipitated by sudden emotional or physical stress. There is growing evidence that exaggerated sympathetic stimulation is central to the pathogenesis of this syndrome. Precisely how catecholamines mediate myocardial stunning in takotsubo syndrome remains incompletely understood; but possible mechanisms include epicardial spasm, microvascular dysfunction, direct adrenergic-receptor–mediated myocyte injury, and systemic vascular effects that alter ventricular-arterial coupling. Risk factors that increase sympathetic tone and/or catecholamine sensitivity may render individuals particularly susceptible to takotsubo syndrome during episodes of acute stress.

Giuseppe Limongelli, Daniele Masarone, Valeria Maddaloni, Marta Rubino, Fiorella Fratta, Annapaola Cirillo, Spinelli Barrile Ludovica, Roberta Pacileo, Adelaide Fusco, Guido Ronald Coppola, Francesca Pisacane, Eduardo Bossone, Paolo Calabrò, Raffaele Calabrò, Maria Giovanna Russo, and Giuseppe Pacileo

Takotsubo syndrome (TTS) is an enigmatic disease with a multifactorial and still unresolved pathogenesis. A genetic predisposition has been suggested based on the few familial TTS cases. Conflicting results have been published regarding the role of functional polymorphisms in relevant candidate genes, such as α_1-, β_1-, and β_2-adrenergic receptors; G protein–coupled receptor kinase 5; and estrogen receptors. Further research is required to help clarify the role of genetic susceptibility in TTS.

Scott W. Sharkey

This article provides a contemporary review of the clinical features of the takotsubo syndrome. It discusses hallmark elements that distinguish this novel acute cardiac condition from the more common acute coronary syndrome. This article includes relevant clinical detail surrounding findings on ECG, biochemical testing, and cardiac imaging and a discussion of complications, including acute decompensated heart failure, arrhythmias, ventricular thrombi, and left ventricular outflow obstruction. The article concludes with discussion of proper treatment, long-term survival, and recurrence.

Influence of Age and Gender in Takotsubo Syndrome

Birke Schneider and Udo Sechtem

Takotsubo syndrome (TTS) occurs predominantly in elderly females but young individuals and children may also be affected. There are no consistent differences between men and women regarding age, symptoms, prehospital delay, or clinical course. Mortality has been reported to be higher in males. The QTc interval may be disproportionately prolonged in male patients in the days after admission predisposing them to ventricular arrhythmias. The higher level of cardiac markers in males with TTS may be related to the greater frequency of physical stress before the onset of TTS. Understanding the pathogenetic background may lead to preventive/therapeutic means against this life-threatening disease.

Chronobiology of Takotsubo Syndrome and Myocardial Infarction: Analogies and Differences

Roberto Manfredini, Fabio Manfredini, Fabio Fabbian, Raffaella Salmi, Massimo Gallerani, Eduardo Bossone, and Abhishek J. Deshmukh

Several pathophysiologic factors, not harmful if taken alone, are capable of triggering unfavorable events when presenting together within the same temporal window (chronorisk), and the occurrence of many cardiovascular events is not evenly distributed in time. Both acute myocardial infarction and takotsubo syndrome seem to exhibit a temporal preference in their onset, characterized by variations according to time of day, day of the week, and month of the year, although with both analogies and differences.

Takotsubo Syndrome and Embolic Events

Ibrahim El-Battrawy, Martin Borggrefe, and Ibrahim Akin

Takotsubo cardiomyopathy (TTC), initially defined as a benign disease, is associated with several complications. One of them is a thromboembolism, which is clinically presented by events such as stroke, ventricular thrombi, and peripheral embolization, and can be present at index event of TCC as well as at any time in disease course. Patients with elevated C-reactive protein levels, markedly elevated D-dimers, and severely impaired left ventricular function seem to be at higher risk of developing thromboemboli. Treatment strategies prescribed in the management of thombembolic complications in patients with acute myocardial infarction includes a short course of anticoagulation. A similar analogy could also be considered for patients with TTC presenting with this complication. Nevertheless, an individualized close-follow-up is of utmost importance to avoid any relapse and not to oversee any impeding complications in light of dynamic processes in myocardial stunning.

Challenges of Chronic Cardiac Problems in Survivors of Takotsubo Syndrome   551

Andrew C. Morley-Smith and Alexander R. Lyon

A hallmark feature of the Takotsubo syndrome (TTS) is the reversible nature of the observed cardiac dysfunction. This is underlined in diagnostic criteria. However, it would appear this reversibility is a subtle process, and that myocardial catecholamine toxicity can cause lasting permanent abnormalities of myocardial physiology. A growing body of evidence suggests persisting abnormalities may predispose post-TTS patients to cardiac and noncardiac morbidity and mortality. The cardiology community needs to understand more clearly how TTS evolves, how to identify high-risk patients with incomplete resolution, and perform studies to assess which treatment(s) are effective to improve cardiac recovery and clinical outcomes.

Contemporary Imaging in Takotsubo Syndrome   559

Rodolfo Citro, Gianluca Pontone, Leonardo Pace, Concetta Zito, Angelo Silverio, Eduardo Bossone, and Federico Piscione

Transthoracic echocardiography is the first-line imaging modality for evaluating patients with Takotsubo syndrome (TTS). Beyond diagnosis, TTE enables detection of peculiar complications and is useful for risk stratification and management of patients with cardiogenic shock. Cardiac magnetic resonance can be used to detect myocardial edema typically associated with TTS and is helpful in the differential diagnosis with other disease states. Coronary computed tomography angiography can be performed as an alternative to coronary angiography to confirm coronary artery patency. Molecular imaging is a promising approach for identifying patients at increased risk of recurrence.

Takotsubo Syndrome—Scientific Basis for Current Treatment Strategies   577

Elmir Omerovic

Takotsubo syndrome (TS) is characterized by severe reversible left ventricular (LV) wall motion abnormality in the absence of explanatory coronary lesion. Despite an increasing number of patients diagnosed with TS worldwide, there are no randomized clinical trials. In mild cases, no treatment or a short course of limited anticoagulation therapy may be sufficient. Positive inotropic and vasodilating agents should be avoided. In severe cases with refractory cardiogenic shock, early treatment with mechanical support using venoarterial extracorporeal membrane oxygenation or a LV assist device should be considered.

Takotsubo Syndrome: Insights from Japan   587

Yoshihiro J. Akashi and Masaharu Ishihara

We report the history and new insights of takotsubo syndrome based on the achievements that Japanese researchers have contributed and summarize the evidence originally presented from Japan. Takotsubo syndrome is a newly described heart failure characterized by transient left ventricular dysfunction. We should be aware of this entity as a syndrome, not actual cardiomyopathy. Japanese researchers focus on the experimental approaches for clinical diagnosis and treatment of takotsubo syndrome. As representatives from a country originally naming this syndrome takotsubo, a global registry for takotsubo syndrome including Japan should be established.

Takotsubo syndrome (TTS) was first described in Japan in 1990. The clinical presentation is similar to that of acute coronary syndrome (ACS). Cardiac enzymes are commonly elevated. A global initiative was launched and the International Takotsubo Registry (InterTAK Registry) was established to provide a systematic database. The major goals of the InterTAK Registry are to provide a comprehensive clinical characterization on natural history, treatment, and outcomes. We linked a biorepository to identify biomarkers for the diagnosis and prognosis and to investigate the genetic basis as well as disease-related factors. We focus on the rationale, objectives, design, and first results of the InterTAK Registry.

HEART FAILURE CLINICS

THE CLINICS ARE AVAILABLE ONLINE!
Access your subscription at:
www.theclinics.com

Preface
Takotsubo: From Cardiomyopathy to Acute Reversible Heart Failure Syndrome

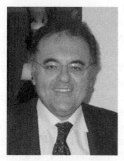

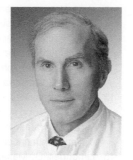

Eduardo Bossone, MD,
PhD, FCCP, FESC, FACC

Raimund Erbel, MD,
FAHA, FESC, FACC, FASE

Editors

Recent multiple registry data and the position statement developed by the Heart Failure Association of the European Society of Cardiology have triggered updating the last *Heart Failure Clinics* issue on Takotsubo syndrome (TTS).[1–6]

HIGHLIGHTS

First, there is a consensus to implement the term "syndrome" instead of cardiomyopathy.[6] Second, a clinical profile (up to 80% of cases) has been depicted.[5] In this regard, it should be underlined that in-hospital and long-term morbidity and mortality are not negligible.[5–10] Coronary angiography and left ventriculography are key tests in the diagnostic pathway of a patient with TTS in order to exclude an acute coronary syndrome.[6] However, an integrated multiimaging approach (first-line two-dimensional transthoracic echocardiography) remains essential to guide therapeutic interventions.[11–13] At the present time, therapy remains empiric and aims to counteract the rapid onset of symptoms and/or signs of heart failure and related

complications. Furthermore, no definite follow-up strategy has been delineated.[14]

CHALLENGES TO BE MET AND OVERCOME

Some of the challenges to be met and overcome include the following:

a. Explore the interplay between genetic susceptibility and pathophysiologic mechanisms.[15–17]
b. Analyze outliers.[18]
c. Implement multiparametric risk scores.[6]
d. Design randomized clinical trials.[6,14]
e. Consider oral anticoagulation treatment.[19]

It is a fascinating journey, please join us and remain updated....

Eduardo Bossone, MD, PhD, FCCP, FESC, FACC
Cardiology Division
"Cava de' Tirreni and Amalfi Coast"
Heart Department, University Hospital
Via De Marinis, 4
84013 Cava de' Tirreni (SA), Italy

Heart Failure Clin 12 (2016) xiii–xiv
http://dx.doi.org/10.1016/j.hfc.2016.08.001
1551-7136/16/© 2016 Published by Elsevier Inc.

heartfailure.theclinics.com

Raimund Erbel, MD, FAHA, FESC, FACC, FASE
Institute of Medical Informatics
Biometry and Epidemiology
University Clinic Essen
Hufelandstrasse 55
D-45147 Essen, Germany

E-mail addresses:
ebossone@hotmail.com (E. Bossone)
erbel@uk-essen.de (R. Erbel)

REFERENCES

1. Bossone E, Erbel R. The "Takotsubo syndrome": from legend to science. Heart Fail Clin 2013;9: xiii–xv.
2. Bossone E, Savarese G, Ferrara F, et al. Takotsubo cardiomyopathy: overview. Heart Fail Clin 2013;9: 249–66.
3. Akashi YJ, Ishihara M. Takotsubo syndrome: insights from Japan. Heart Fail Clin, in press.
4. Ghadri JR, Cammann VL, Templin C. The International Takotsubo Registry: rationale, design, objectives, and first results. Heart Fail Clin, in press.
5. Templin C, Ghadri JR, Diekmann J, et al. Clinical features and outcomes of Takotsubo (stress) cardiomyopathy. N Engl J Med 2015;373:929–38.
6. Lyon AR, Bossone E, Schneider B, et al. Current state of knowledge on Takotsubo syndrome: a position statement from the Taskforce on Takotsubo Syndrome of the Heart Failure Association of the European Society of Cardiology. Eur J Heart Fail 2016;18:8–27.
7. Sharkey SW. A clinical perspective of the Takotsubo syndrome. Heart Fail Clin, in press.
8. Schneider B, Sechtem U. Influence of age and gender in Takotsubo syndrome. Heart Fail Clin, in press.
9. Manfredini R, Manfredini F, Fabbian F, et al. Chronobiology of Takotsubo syndrome and myocardial infarction: analogies and differences. Heart Fail Clin, in press.
10. Morley-Smith AC, Lyon AR. Challenges of chronic cardiac problems in survivors of Takotsubo syndrome. Heart Fail Clin, in press.
11. Bossone E, Lyon A, Citro R, et al. Takotsubo cardiomyopathy: an integrated multi-imaging approach. Eur Heart J Cardiovasc Imaging 2014;15:366–77.
12. Citro R, Rigo F, D'Andrea A, et al. Echocardiographic correlates of acute heart failure, cardiogenicshock, and in-hospital mortality in tako-tsubo cardiomyopathy. JACC Cardiovasc Imaging 2014;7:119–29.
13. Citro R, Pontone G, Pace L, et al. Contemporary imaging in Takotsubo syndrome. Heart Fail Clin, in press.
14. Omerovic E. Takotsubo syndrome: scientific basis for current treatment strategies. Heart Fail Clin, in press.
15. Limongelli G, Masarone D, Maddaloni V, et al. Genetics of Takotsubo syndrome. Heart Fail Clin, in press.
16. Williams R, Arri S, Prasad A. Current concepts in the pathogenesis of Takotsubo syndrome. Heart Fail Clin, in press.
17. Wittstein IS. The sympathetic nervous system in the pathogenesis of Takotsubo syndrome. Heart Fail Clin, in press.
18. Maseri A. New targets for prevention: identification of specific disease mechanisms. G Ital Cardiol (Rome) 2009;10(11-12 Suppl 3):39S–42S.
19. El-Battrawy I, Behnes M, Borggrefe M, et al. Takotsubo syndrome and embolic events. Heart Fail Clin, in press.

Current Concepts in the Pathogenesis of Takotsubo Syndrome

Rupert Williams, MBBS, MRCP, PhD[a,1],
Satpal Arri, MBBS, MRCP[b,1],
Abhiram Prasad, MD, FRCP, FACC, FESC[a,*]

KEYWORDS

- Takotsubo syndrome • Apical ballooning syndrome • Catecholamine • Pathophysiology

KEY POINTS

- The pathophysiology of Takotsubo syndrome (TTS) seems to be complex and likely includes exaggerated cardiovascular responses to surges in catecholamine levels.
- Patients with TTS have a high burden of premorbid psychiatric and neurologic diseases.
- Impaired vascular function, especially of the microcirculation, seems to be a common feature.
- Ventricular dysfunction seen in TTS may represent a form of protective stunning with downregulation of noncritical cellular functions, thus preventing cellular necrosis.

INTRODUCTION

Despite 25 years of extensive efforts to characterize the underlying pathophysiology of Takotsubo syndrome (TTS), current knowledge remains limited.[1–3] The initial presentation, both clinically and electrocardiographically, is similar to an acute myocardial infarction (AMI).[4,5] The biomarker profile is also similar,[4] although the peak troponin and creatinine kinase levels are lower, and brain natriuretic peptide levels are higher in patients with TTS compared with ST-segment elevation AMI.[5] TTS occurs most frequently in women (ratio 9:1),[4,6,7] particularly postmenopausal women. Most cases are triggered by an emotional or physical stressor, although in around 30% of patients no trigger is identified.[4] TTS culminates in an acute heart failure syndrome with a prognosis that is perhaps worse than had been previously thought;

the largest international registry recently reported similar in-hospital rates of cardiogenic shock and mortality to those of patients with an AMI.[4]

This article reviews the leading hypotheses for the pathophysiology of TTS, which is seemingly complex, and likely includes exaggerated cardiovascular responses, in susceptible individuals, to stress and surges in catecholamine levels.

CATECHOLAMINE HYPOTHESIS

The temporal relationship between stressful triggers, along with several documented cases of TTS triggered by iatrogenic catecholamines, suggests a central role for the adrenergic system in the pathophysiology. As such, β-blockers have been proposed as a treatment to prevent recurrence,[8] although clinical trials have not been conducted.

Disclosure: The authors have nothing to disclose.
[a] Cardiovascular and Cell Sciences Research Institute, St. George's, University of London, Cranmer Terrace, London SW17 0RE, UK; [b] Cardiovascular Division, Rayne Institute, King's College London, St Thomas' Hospital, Westminster Bridge Road, London SE1 7EH, UK
[1] Equal contribution.
* Corresponding author.
E-mail address: aprasad@sgul.ac.uk

Heart Failure Clin 12 (2016) 473–484
http://dx.doi.org/10.1016/j.hfc.2016.06.002
1551-7136/16/$ – see front matter © 2016 Elsevier Inc. All rights reserved.

Animal Models

Rapid and extreme increases in systolic and diastolic blood pressure, associated with acute reversible apical hypokinesia, have been reported to develop within minutes following intraperitoneal or intravenous catecholamine administration in several animal models.[9–13] In some experiments, the severity of hypokinesia has been sufficient to cause cardiogenic shock.[14] In a primate model, coadministration of metoprolol resulted in slight amelioration of left ventricular (LV) systolic impairment and reduction of cardiomyocytolysis.[8] Multiple catecholamines, including epinenephrine,[12,14] norepinephrine,[12] dopamine,[12] phenylephrine,[12] and isoprenaline,[12,13,15] have been shown to induce apical hypokinesis. There is apparent heterogeneity in these animal models depending on the type of catecholamine used and the route of administration.

In addition to exogenous catecholamine administration, emotional stress in rats induced by immobilization has also been shown to induce reversible apical hypokinesis.[16] These effects were normalized pretreatment with amosulalol hydrochloride, an αβ-adrenoceptor blocker. Although these animal models provide a much-needed opportunity to investigate the pathophysiology of TTS, their reproducibility and relevance to the clinical condition remain to be established.

The mechanisms by which regional, rather than global, wall motion abnormalities are induced are not immediately evident. One explanation for this phenomenon is that there may be regional heterogeneity in catecholamine sensitivity.[12,17] It has been reported that the canine left ventricle has an apex to base gradient of beta-adrenergic receptors (β-ARs), with an increased density at the apex.[12] The differential distribution may be present to maintain the apical contribution to LV ejection during acute stress. In contrast, sympathetic nerve density is lowest in the apex of the canine heart (and highest in the base) and this may offset any differences resulting from the β-AR gradient.[12] However, it is unknown whether similar β-AR and nerve density gradients are present in the human heart.

A potential unifying hypothesis that has been proposed is related to the different mechanisms for norepinephrine and epinephrine release. Norepinephrine is predominantly released from sympathetic neurons, which potentially have their highest density at the base of the ventricle, whereas epinephrine is predominantly a circulating catecholamine derived from the adrenal gland[18] Thus, following a major stressful trigger, there would be predominant basal norepinephrine stimulation and apical epinephrine effect caused by the higher density of β-ARs (**Fig. 1**).[12]

Another hypothesis proposes that it may be catecholaminergic stimulation of pleiotropic β_2-adrenoceptors, which is particularly important in inducing TTS by mediating a signaling switch from cardiostimulation to cardioinhibition pathways, via activation of Gi instead of Gs proteins.[14,19,20] This process is referred to as stimulus trafficking and is thought to occur at very high concentrations of epinephrine, resulting in a negative inotropic stimulus.

There are limitations to the current knowledge from animal models. For example, the effects of repeated administration of low doses of exogenous catecholamine are unclear.[13,14] Published studies have focused on the effects of catecholamine toxicity and may not be representative of the human condition.[21] Further studies are needed to understand the role of the autonomic nervous system in TTS, and with that knowledge design animal models that may be more representative.

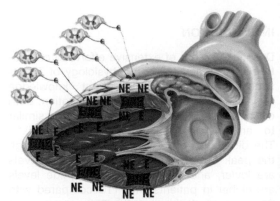

Fig. 1. Excess regional cardiac catecholamine release. Epinephrine (E) and norepinephrine (NE) are released from nonneural local stores within the myocardium (*blue areas*). Local concentrations of catecholamine are thought to differ between different myocardial regions because of heterogeneities in sympathetic nerve innervation and local intramyocardial stores. NE dominates among the catecholamine released from sympathetic nerve endings, whereas E dominates among catecholamine released from local stores. Hence, NE predominates in basal regions and E predominates in apical regions. These heterogeneities may translate to changes in adrenoceptor density and/or sensitivity as well as alterations in downstream signaling pathways. (*From* Redfors B, Shao Y, Ali A, et al. Current hypotheses regarding the pathophysiology behind the takotsubo syndrome. Int J Cardiol 2014;177(3):775; with permission.)

Human Studies

A TTS-like cardiomyopathy has been described secondary to norepinephrine-secreting, dopamine-secreting, and most commonly epinephrine-secreting pheochromocytomas.[22,23] These cases, together with reports of TTS induced by deliberate or accidental administration of high doses of catecholamines, also support a central role of the sympathetic nervous system in the pathophysiology (Table 1).[24,25] Mental stress has been shown to reduce LV ejection fraction, and, rarely, induces regional wall motion abnormalities in conjunction with an increase in catecholamine levels.[26]

Very high circulating blood levels of epinephrine and norepinephrine at the time of TTS presentation, persisting over a period of several days, were reported in one study.[27] However, this has not been a consistent finding, with several studies reporting normal catecholamine levels,[28,29] although these studies have been limited in that they measured catecholamines at 1 time point. A study from the Mayo Clinic found 24-hour urine levels of fractionated catecholamines and metanephrines to be normal.[30]

Histology

Two studies of endomyocardial biopsies in patients with TTS have been performed to date[31,32] and these have shown findings to be similar to those associated with catecholamine toxicity of pheochromocytoma and subarachnoid hemorrhage, albeit in very small numbers of patients.[33,34] Abnormalities detected on electron microscopy include the following[31]:

1. An increased diameter of cardiomyocytes caused by the appearance of intracellular vacuoles filled with myelin bodies and cellular debris
2. Disarray of cytoskeletal and contractile proteins
3. Contraction bands consistent with cytoplasmic calcium overload and myofilament cross-bridging
4. Expansion of the extracellular matrix with fibrotic material collagen fibrils and myofibroblasts

Repeat endomyocardial biopsies taken from the same location following recovery of LV ejection fraction showed normal-sized cardiomyocytes with only a few vacuoles and normal extracellular matrix.

Immunohistochemistry findings include (Fig. 2)[31,32]:

1. Structural disarrangement of intracellular proteins (alpha-actinin, actin, and titin)[31]
2. Expansion of the extracellular matrix with increased levels of collagen-I,[31] and increased

ratio of collagen-I to collagen-III (a marker of elasticity)[32]
3. High transforming growth factor-beta levels, stimulating secretion of connective tissue growth factors and profibrotic osteopontin.[32]

Endomyocardial biopsies taken following LV functional recovery show a normal arrangement of intracellular proteins, and a reduction in collagen-I deposition (although it is increased compared with reference samples) and fibrosis.[31] It is hypothesized that the magnitude of myocardial fibrosis is not sufficient to irreversibly damage structural integrity, therefore allowing functional recovery.[29,31] Furthermore, it is suggested that myofibroblasts may protect against irreversible damage by mitigating myocardial disarray.[31]

These histologic changes may represent the sequelae of high concentrations of intracellular calcium (mediated via cyclic AMP, through interference with sodium and calcium channel transporters following free radical damage).[27,31,33] Intracellular calcium overload is thought to have a causal role in ventricular dysfunction induced by catecholamine toxicity.[34]

HYPOTHALAMIC-PITUITARY-ADRENAL AXIS HYPOTHESIS

Animal experiments suggest that the hypothalamic-pituitary-adrenal axis (HPAA) may contribute to TTS. Steroid pretreatment predisposes animals to cardiac contraction band necrosis and a cardiomyopathy when exposed to a variety of stressors.[35] Madhavan and colleagues[30] reported that evening plasma cortisol levels are increased during acute TTS presentation, but no greater in magnitude than those seen in a control group with ST elevation AMI. Twenty-four-hour urine free cortisol levels were normal, suggesting that the activation of the corticosteroid system is not sustained beyond the acute period.

Salivary cortisol responses have been investigated in 19 female patients with TTS after recovery and compared with controls with a prior myocardial infarction and healthy women.[36] Basal physiologic function of the HPAA was not different between the groups, but patients with TTS tended to have a blunted cortisol stress response. These data are in keeping with previous observations of hyporesponsiveness (hypocortisolism) of the HPAA in patients with a history of stress-related diseases, such as chronic fatigue syndrome,[37] fibromyalgia,[38] and posttraumatic stress disorder.[39] It is hypothesized that this is a consequence of chronic HPAA activation.[40]

Table 1
Data on epinephrine administration-triggered Takotsubo syndrome in 22 patients

N	Age (y)	Female	Dose (mg)	Route	Circumstances
1	37	1	0.9	IV	Administered for anaphylaxis
1	67	0	<3.2[b]	Topical	Administered for maxillary surgery
1	49	1	0.1 × 3	IV	Administered for anaphylaxis
1	44	1	0.3 + 3.0	SC	Second dose given inadvertently for drug anaphylaxis
1	44	1	1.0	IV	Administered for contrast anaphylaxis for CTA
1	26	1	0.5	IM	Administered for anaphylaxis
1	81	0	0.3/1.0	IM/IV	Administered for anaphylaxis
1	50	1	0.5	IV	Administered for anaphylaxis during anesthesia
1	55	1	NS	IV	Administered for anaphylaxis during anesthesia
1	37	1	1.0	IV	Administered for anaphylaxis
1	39	1	1.0	IV	Inadvertently injected during an ACTH stimulation test
1	70	1	0.3	IV	Administered for anaphylaxis
1	61	1	High-dose EN	IV	Administered for anaphylaxis during anesthesia
1	31	1	NS; 1:10^5	SM	Administered for nasal sinus surgery
1	59	0	0.04	SM	Administered for ethmoid sinus surgery
1	41	1	1.0	IV	Larger dose was administered inadvertently for anaphylaxis
1	27	0	2.0	IV	Self-administered; history of drug abuse
1	24	1	5.0	IM	Administered inadvertently for anaphylaxis
1	76	1	0.3[a]	IM	Self-administered for generalized urticaria and oral angioedema
1	36	1	NS	SC	Administered for ear plastic surgery
1	62	0	2.4	SC	Self-administered 0.3 mg × 8 over 4 h for asthma exacerbation
1	48	1	NS	IM/LCIR	Local irrigation for shoulder arthroscopy
Total = 22	48.4 ± 16.3	17	(72.3%)	Dose 1.4 ± 1.4 mg	

Abbreviations: ACTH, adrenocorticotropic hormone; CTA, computed tomography angiography; EN, epinephrine and norepinephrine infused intravenously; IM, intramuscular; IV, intravenous; LCIR, local continuous irrigation; NS, amount not specified; SC, subcutaneous; SM, submucosal.

[a] The patient was on oxprenolol 20 mg daily, a medication with intrinsic sympathomimetic activity, which, with its partial agonist effect, may have paradoxically perpetuated the catecholamine effects.

[b] The surplus was suctioned from the nasopharynx after removal of the pads.

From Madias JE. Epinephrine administration and Takotsubo syndrome: lessons from past experiences. Int J Carciol 2016;207:101; with permission.

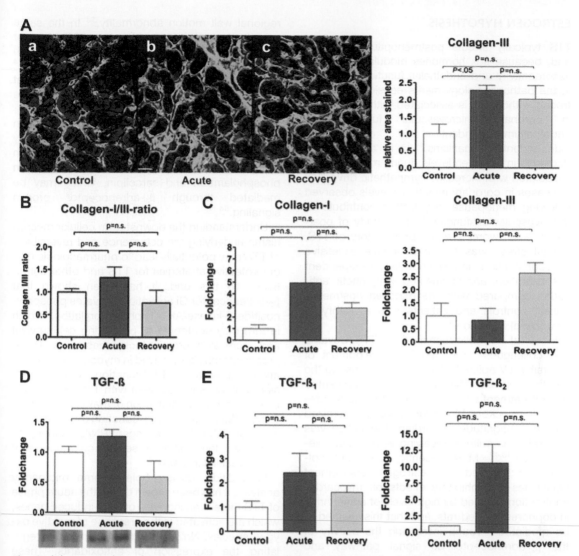

Fig. 2. (A) Immunohistochemical staining for extracellular matrix proteins. Collagen-III (*green*), nuclei (*blue*, Draq5TM), and f-actin (*red*, Phalloidin – tetramethylrhodamine B isothiocyanate conjugate [TRTC]). Compared with controls, collagen-III significantly accumulates between cardiomyocytes in biopsies from acute TTS and consecutively widens the interstitial space. After functional recovery, collagen-III content decreases, but remains greater than values of healthy controls. (B) Considering results for collagen-I, a shift in the collagen-I/collagen-III ratio could be documented. (C) Quantitative real-time polymerase chain reaction showed an increased expression of collagen-I in acute samples with a decline after functional recovery. Expression levels of collagen-III were not altered in the acute phase but revealed an increase in recovery samples. (D) Western blot analysis revealed an increased amount of the protein transforming growth factor-beta (TGF-β) in acute TTS with consecutive decline after recovery of functional LV parameters. (E) Accordingly, quantitative real-time reverse transcription polymerase chain reaction analysis showed an increased transcriptional rate for messenger RNA of TGF-β1 and TGF-β2. (*From* Szardien S, Möllmann H, Willmer M, et al. Molecular basis of disturbed extracellular matrix homeostasis in stress cardiomyopathy. Int J Cardiol 2013;168(2):1686; with permission.)

Studies in animals[41] and humans[42] have shown suppression of catecholamine turnover with glucocorticoid release. Lower levels of cortisol release in response to a mental stressor have also been associated with greater negative emotional arousal, preventing so-called emotional homeostasis after mental stress.[43] Thus, hypocortisolism during stressful triggers may prevent the important inhibitory influence of cortisol on catecholamine release, a process that potentially could contribute to the pathophysiology of TTS.

ESTROGEN HYPOTHESIS

TTS typically affects postmenopausal women, and, because sex hormones modulate coronary vasoreactivity and endothelial function, their role in the pathophysiology merits consideration. Estrogen withdrawal is associated with impairment in coronary microvascular function via endothelium-dependent and endothelium-independent mechanisms.[44,45] In addition, the decrease in estrogen levels during menopause is associated with increased sympathetic drive.[44,45] Increases in coronary endothelin levels observed following menopause may further contribute to microvascular dysfunction.[46] In a study of post-menopausal women with a prior history of TTS, mental stress was shown to induce excessive vasoconstriction, impair endothelium-dependent vasodilatation, and augmented sympathetic activation compared with age matched postmenopausal controls and patients with a history of myocardial infarction.[47]

In the rat immobilization model of TTS, Ueyama and colleagues[48] reported the development of reversible LV apical ballooning in response to the emotional stress. This ballooning was prevented by pretreatment with α-adrenoceptor and β-adrenoceptor blockers. Moreover, in oophorectomized rats, the magnitude of cardiac dysfunction was diminished in animals receiving estrogen supplementation.[48,49] More recently, Cao and colleagues[50] showed that estrogen replacement diminishes the inhibitory effects on myocardial contraction induced by high levels of epinephrine in oophorectomized rats, and that this seemed to be mediated through increasing the activity of the β_2-adrenoceptor–Gs signal pathway and decreasing the concentration of catecholamine in plasma.

Additional potential reasons for a pathophysiologic role for sex hormones include the expression of estrogen receptor on cardiac myocytes, which may modulate cardiac contractility[51]; and the regulation of calcium uptake in myocytes.[52]

CELL SIGNALING

The most widely discussed cell signaling hypothesis is the switch from β_2-adrenoceptor Gs to Gi protein at very high concentrations of epinephrine,[14,53] although this remains controversial and needs confirmation.[12] The hypothesis proposes that activation of Gi protein reduces cyclic AMP levels (in contrast with Gs protein activation), thereby reducing inotropy. In the animal model, pretreatment with the pertussis toxin, an inhibitor of Gi signaling, prevented epinephrine-mediated

regional wall motion abnormality.[14] In the same model norepinephrine, which has 20-fold lower affinity for β_2-adrenoceptors compared with β_1-adrenoceptors, was unable to produce TTS,[14] although other investigators have reported that both epinephrine and norepinephrine can induce TTS-like cardiac dysfunction.[12]

Sarcoplasmic/endoplasmic reticulum calcium ATPase (SERCA2) has been shown to be markedly inhibited in the acute phase of TTS through upregulation of the intrinsic membrane protein phospholamban and sarcolipin, which may be mediated through β_1-adrenoceptor protein signaling.[54]

Understanding the downstream cellular mechanisms underlying the occurrence and reversibility of TTS may potentially lead to pharmacologic cardioprotective strategies for TTS and other conditions. To this end, it has been shown that β_2-adrenoceptor Gi activation activates phosphoinositide 3 kinase/AKT-1 phosphorylation, which in turn may contribute to promoting cell survival and increasing protein biosynthesis.[29,55] These processes may be involved in myocardial regeneration and recovery of LV function. Rapid regression of fibrosis is also seen with TTS, which may be mediated via upregulation of matrix metalloproteinase (MMP)-9, through reduction of tissue inhibitors of MMP-3 messenger RNA, leading to increased degradation of several components of the extracellular matrix.[32]

In addition, using whole-genome microarray analysis, it has been shown that in the acute phase of TTS there is an increase of Nrf2-induced genes, which are activated in the presence of reactive oxygen species. Nrf2 is a transcription factor regulating the expression of antioxidants. These findings link catecholamine excess with oxidative stress in TTS. During recovery, there is upregulation of genes involved in energy, fatty acid, and carbohydrate metabolism, perhaps reflecting mechanisms leading to contractile recovery.[56]

GENETICS AND TAKOTSUBO SYNDROME

The possibility of a genetic underpinning of TTS is raised by a small number of familial cases reported in the literature.[57–59] This is further supported by reports of α-adrenoceptor and β-adrenoceptor polymorphisms being associated with the risk of cardiac injury and dysfunction in patients with subarachnoid haemorrhage,[60] a condition well known to lead to TTS/neurogenic stunned myocardium. Genetic studies in TTS have yielded variable results. Sharkey and colleagues[61] reported no difference in adrenoceptor ADRA2C and ADRB1 polymorphisms in TTS versus controls. In contrast,

Vriz and colleagues[62] found differences in β1 (Arg389Gly; homozygous Arg/Arg more frequent in TTS), and β2-adrenoreceptor (Gln27Glu; homozygous Gln/Gln less frequent in TTS) polymorphisms, but no difference at β2-adrenoreceptor (Arg16Gly) polymorphism. In addition, another study explored several polymorphisms in the adrenergic system and found no major difference except for a higher prevalence among TTS of the polymorphism Q41L in the G-protein–coupled receptor kinase 5 genes,[63] a variant with putative negative inotropic effects under conditions of acute catecholamine stimulation.

A major limitation of these gene-targeted studies is an incomplete genetic characterization of the complex adrenergic signaling network. In order to overcome this, Goodloe and colleagues[64] conducted whole-exome sequencing to characterize genetic variation of the adrenergic signaling pathways. Analysis of common functional adrenergic polymorphisms identified no differences in functional allele frequency or burden between TTS and healthy controls, including in a mother-daughter pair. Moreover, the findings reported by Vriz and colleagues[62] and Spinelli and colleagues[63] were not replicated in this cohort.

PSYCHOLOGICAL FACTORS AND PERSONALITY

Patients diagnosed with TTS are more likely to have a premorbid diagnosis of a chronic anxiety disorder compared with age-matched and gender-matched acute coronary syndrome and general population controls.[65,66] They are also more likely to have a family history of anxiety or depression and more likely to report social stressors such as being divorced and isolated. These observations from small single-center studies have been replicated in a large international multicenter registry of 1750 patients with TTS in which approximately 30% of patients had a history of a prior or chronic psychiatric disorder, which is more than 2-fold higher than a control population of patients with acute coronary syndrome.[4] Similarly, there was a higher prevalence of chronic neurologic disorders, suggesting a link between neuropsychiatric disorders and TTS.

An interesting association is that patients with TTS seem to have a higher frequency of migraine and Raynaud phenomenon.[67] TTS, migraine, and Raynaud share characteristics such as female predominance, precipitation by triggers, altered vascular reactivity, and increased likelihood of associated affective disorders. Patients with migraine and Raynaud who have no diagnosis of affective disorders have been reported to have greater neuroticism, a normal personality trait defined as a propensity to experience negative affect that is expressed as nervousness and insecurity.[68,69] However, a recent study in TTS found that these patients did not manifest higher levels of neuroticism and do not have greater vulnerability to stress than the general population.[70]

In contrast, Compare and colleagues[71] proposed that patients who experience emotionally triggered TTS have a higher frequency of type D personality compared with those without emotional triggering. Type D (distressed) personality is characterized by high negative affectivity (tendency to experience negative emotions) and high social inhibition (tendency to inhibit the expression of emotions/behaviors in social interactions to avoid disapproval). In addition, Del Pace and colleagues[72] evaluated the presence of high-anxiety trait in patients with TTS compared with age-matched, gender-matched, and hypertension-matched patients with ST-elevation myocardial infarction. High-anxiety trait was common in patients with TTS, but no different from patients who had sustained a myocardial infarction.

MYOCARDIAL ISCHEMIA AND INCREASED WALL STRESS
Coronary Microvascular Dysfunction

Microvascular dysfunction is frequently detected at presentation in Takotsubo syndrome
TIMI frame count, an angiographic measure of coronary blood flow, is reversibly prolonged in all 3 major epicardial coronary vessels.[73,74] Elesber and colleagues[75] observed abnormal microvascular perfusion in approximately two-thirds of cases using myocardial blush grading, another angiographic measure of perfusion. There was a correlation between the magnitude of troponin level increase and electrocardiogram abnormalities with the severity of microvascular dysfunction. Kume and colleagues[76] reported a decrease in coronary flow reserve in all 3 coronary arteries using Doppler flow wire, and others have done the same noninvasively with Doppler transthoracic echocardiography.[77] The microcirculatory disturbances may recover at around day 7, paralleling contractile recovery.[77]

Single-photon emission computed tomography using thallium and sestamibi tracers, and PET using 13N-ammonia, have consistently shown impaired perfusion in the regions of the wall motion abnormality.[73,78,79] The reduction in myocardial fatty acid and glucose metabolism in the acute phase tends to be greater than the reduction in myocardial perfusion.[80,81] The authors speculate that the ventricular dysfunction represents a form of protective stunning with downregulation of noncritical cellular functions, thus preventing cellular necrosis,[12] akin to ischemic preconditioning.[82] At this time, it is unknown whether the impairment in microvascular function is the primary mechanism for the injury or an epiphenomenon. Potential reasons for this being a secondary process include that the myocardial edema, frequently present in akinetic regions, can impair microvascular function.[83] Moreover, in a rat model there was no regional perfusion abnormality observed before the development of LV dysfunction.[84] In contrast, a primary pathophysiologic role is supported by the findings of Patel and colleagues,[85] conducted many months after recovery from TTS, in which most patients had abnormal coronary microvascular function in response to either acetylcholine and/or adenosine, and this was often severe.

Multivessel Coronary Spasm

Patients with TTS typically present with chest pain and ischemic changes on the electrocardiogram that mimic an AMI.[86] Early reported cases were associated with multivessel coronary spasm at angiography, leading investigators to postulate this as the mechanism for myocardial stunning.[1] However, in a subsequent larger case series, spontaneous coronary spasm was only reported in approximately 10% of patients.[2,74] It is possible that the routine administration of nitrates for ischemic chest pain in current treatment pathways may obscure the presence of spasm by the time an angiogram is performed. However, less than a third of patients showed inducible coronary spasm following ergonovine or acetylcholine provocation testing, and the clinical relevance of this finding is questionable, because endothelial dysfunction is highly prevalent in postmenopausal women, and suggests that other mechanisms are likely at play. High levels of endothelin, a potent vasoconstrictor, have been measured in patients with acute TTS, but again this is of uncertain clinical significance.[87]

Spontaneously Aborted Myocardial Infarction

Spontaneous thrombolysis following acute plaque rupture and transient occlusive thrombus has also been postulated as a potential mechanism of TTS.[3] Ibanez and colleagues[88] observed ruptured plaques on intravascular ultrasonography (IVUS) imaging of the left anterior descending artery (LAD) in patients with TTS. The investigators postulated that TTS results from an aborted anterior AMI in patients with a long wrap-around LAD.[88] However, this has not been a reproducible finding and others have failed to show culprit lesions using IVUS, and in one series less than a third of patients with TTS had a long wrap-around LAD.[89,90]

The extent of regional wall motion abnormality and the magnitude of LV systolic impairment is unlikely to be accounted for by transient interruption of flow by spasm or occlusive thrombus in a single epicardial coronary artery. Simultaneous spasm affecting left and right coronary arteries or multivessel thrombi affecting the entire apical and midventricular vascular bed is unlikely. Furthermore, the female preponderance of the condition is in contrast with the predilection of coronary atherosclerosis in men. Almost all patients with TTS either have angiographically normal coronary arteries or mild atherosclerosis. Obstructive coronary artery disease may coexist by virtue of its prevalence in the population at risk.[90]

Left Ventricular Outflow Tract Obstruction

LV outflow tract obstruction may be detected in up to 25% of patients, and has been associated with LV septal bulge and systolic anterior motion of the mitral valve.[91] This finding has led some investigators to hypothesize that TTS could be a consequence of severe transient LV outflow tract obstruction resulting from hyperkinesis induced by intense catecholamine stimulation.[92]

LV wall stress is distributed evenly in the normal heart. During acute TTS, LV end-systolic pressure and wall stress can increase significantly.[93] Significant systemic hypertension has been reported in patients with pheochromocytoma and following a subarachnoid hemorrhage. This hypertension can be transient with subsequent hypotension and the resulting typical apical dysfunction.[94] This finding has led to the suggestion that excess cardiac stimulation in the setting of hypotension may redistribute wall tension toward the apical segments.[95]

In a rat model, intraperitoneal administration of isoprenaline has been shown to reduce blood pressure and produce a typical apical variant of TTS.[95] Thus, Redfors and colleagues[95] speculated that the combination of a low afterload and high inotropic drive may obliterate the LV cavity during systole, resulting in transient outflow tract obstruction and excessive apical wall stress. When phenylephrine was coadministered to maintain systolic blood pressure (120–160 mm Hg) cardiac dysfunction was not seen. In contrast, primary vasoconstrictors, such as epinephrine, norepinephrine, and dopamine, increased afterload, and resulted in the basal Takotsubo variant.[95] Furthermore, coadministration of vasodilators decreased the incidence of atypical LV dysfunction and instead the rats were more likely to develop typical apical dysfunction.[95]

SUMMARY

There has been significant progress made toward understanding the pathophysiology of TTS over the past decade. Although there is no single unifying hypothesis, there is an emerging understanding of the interplay between the sympathetic nervous system, impaired coronary perfusion, and specific predisposing comorbid conditions. Ongoing research will lead to refinement of the hypotheses discussed.

REFERENCES

1. Dote K, Sato H, Tateishi H, et al. Myocardial stunning due to simultaneous multivessel coronary spasms: a review of 5 cases. J Cardiol 1991;21(2):203–14.
2. Bybee KA, Kara T, Prasad A, et al. Systematic review: transient left ventricular apical ballooning: a syndrome that mimics ST-segment elevation myocardial infarction. Ann Intern Med 2004; 141(11):858–65.
3. Prasad A, Lerman A, Rihal CS. Apical ballooning syndrome (Tako-Tsubo or stress cardiomyopathy): a mimic of acute myocardial infarction. Am Heart J 2008;155(3):408–17.
4. Templin C, Ghadri JR, Diekmann J, et al. Clinical features and outcomes of Takotsubo (stress) cardiomyopathy. N Engl J Med 2015;373(10):929–38.
5. Ahmed KA, Madhavan M, Prasad A. Brain natriuretic peptide in apical ballooning syndrome (Takotsubo/stress cardiomyopathy). Coron Artery Dis 2012; 23(4):259–64.
6. Sharkey SW, Windenburg DC, Lesser JR, et al. Natural history and expansive clinical profile of stress (Tako-Tsubo) cardiomyopathy. J Am Coll Cardiol 2010;55(4):333–41.
7. Schneider B, Athanasiadis A, Stollberger C, et al. Gender differences in the manifestation of tako-tsubo cardiomyopathy. Int J Cardiol 2013;166(3):584–8.
8. Izumi Y, Okatani H, Shiota M, et al. Effects of metoprolol on epinephrine-induced takotsubo-like left ventricular dysfunction in non-human primates. Hypertens Res 2009;32(5):339–46.
9. Mori H, Ishikawa S, Kojima S, et al. Increased responsiveness of left ventricular apical myocardium to adrenergic stimuli. Cardiovasc Res 1993; 27(2):192–8.
10. Lathers CM, Levin RM, Spivey WH. Regional distribution of myocardial beta-adrenoceptors in the cat. Eur J Pharmacol 1986;130(1–2):111–7.
11. Mantravadi R, Gabris B, Liu T, et al. Autonomic nerve stimulation reverses ventricular repolarization sequence in rabbit hearts. Circ Res 2007;100(7): e72–80.
12. Redfors B, Shao Y, Ali A, et al. Current hypotheses regarding the pathophysiology behind the takotsubo syndrome. Int J Cardiol 2014;177(3):771–9.
13. Shao Y, Redfors B, Scharin Täng M, et al. Novel rat model reveals important roles of β-adrenoreceptors in stress-induced cardiomyopathy. Int J Cardiol 2013;168(3):1943–50.
14. Paur H, Wright PT, Sikkel MB, et al. High levels of circulating epinephrine trigger apical cardiodepression in a β 2-adrenergic receptor/Gi-dependent manner: a new model of takotsubo cardiomyopathy. Circulation 2012;126(6):697–706.
15. Heather LC, Catchpole AF, Stuckey DJ, et al. Isoproterenol induces in vivo functional and metabolic abnormalities; similar to those found in the infarcted rat heart. J Physiol Pharmacol 2009;60(3):31–9.
16. Ueyama T, Kasamatsu K, Hano T, et al. Emotional stress induces transient left ventricular hypocontraction in the rat via activation of cardiac adrenoceptors: a possible animal model of "tako-tsubo" cardiomyopathy. Circ J 2002;66(7):712–3.
17. Habecker BA, Malec NM, Landis SC. Differential regulation of adrenergic receptor development by sympathetic innervation. J Neurosci 1996;16(1): 229–37.
18. Kume T, Kawamoto T, Okura H, et al. Local release of catecholamines from the hearts of patients with tako-tsubo-like left ventricular dysfunction. Circ J 2008;72(1):106–8.
19. Wang Y, De Arcangelis V, Gao X, et al. Norepinephrine- and epinephrine-induced distinct beta2-adrenoceptor signaling is dictated by GRK2 phosphorylation in cardiomyocytes. J Biol Chem 2008;283(4):1799–807.
20. Heubach JF, Ravens U, Kaumann AJ. Epinephrine activates both Gs and Gi pathways, but norepinephrine activates only the Gs pathway through human 2-adrenoceptors overexpressed in mouse heart. Mol Pharmacol 2004;65(5):1313–22.
21. Madias JE. Plausible speculations on the pathophysiology of Takotsubo syndrome. Int J Cardiol 2015;188(1):19–21.
22. Lenders J, Eisenhofer G, Mannelli M, et al. Phaeochromocytoma. Lancet 2005;366(9486):665–75.
23. Zielen P, Klisiewicz A, Januszewicz A, et al. Pheochromocytoma-related "classic" takotsubo cardiomyopathy. J Hum Hypertens 2010;24(5):363–6.
24. Abraham J, Mudd JO, Kapur N, et al. Stress cardiomyopathy after intravenous administration of catecholamines and beta-receptor agonists. J Am Coll Cardiol 2009;53(15):1320–5.
25. Ono R, Falcão LM. Takotsubo cardiomyopathy systematic review: pathophysiologic process, clinical

presentation and diagnostic approach to Takotsubo cardiomyopathy. Int J Cardiol 2016;209:196–205.

26. Becker LC, Pepine CJ, Bonsall R, et al. Left ventricular, peripheral vascular, and neurohumoral responses to mental stress in normal middle-aged men and women. Reference Group for the Psychophysiological Investigations of Myocardial Ischemia (PIMI) Study. Circulation 1996;94(11):2768–77.

27. Wittstein IS, Thiemann DR, Lima JA, et al. Neurohumoral features of myocardial stunning due to sudden emotional stress. N Engl J Med 2005;352: 539–48.

28. Y-Hassan S, Henareh L. Plasma catecholamine levels in patients with takotsubo syndrome: implications for the pathogenesis of the disease. Int J Cardiol 2015;181:35–8.

29. Akashi YJ, Nef HM, Lyon AR. Epidemiology and pathophysiology of Takotsubo syndrome. Nat Rev Cardiol 2015;12(7):387–97.

30. Madhavan M, Borlaug BA, Lerman A, et al. Stress hormone and circulating biomarker profile of apical ballooning syndrome (Takotsubo cardiomyopathy): insights into the clinical significance of B-type natriuretic peptide and troponin levels. Heart 2009; 95(17):1436–41.

31. Nef HM, Möllmann H, Kostin S, et al. Tako-Tsubo cardiomyopathy: intraindividual structural analysis in the acute phase and after functional recovery. Eur Heart J 2007;28(20):2456–64.

32. Szardien S, Möllmann H, Willmer M, et al. Molecular basis of disturbed extracellular matrix homeostasis in stress cardiomyopathy. Int J Cardiol 2013; 168(2):1685–8.

33. Wybraniec M, Mizia-Stec K, Krzych Ł. Neurocardiogenic injury in subarachnoid hemorrhage: a wide spectrum of catecholamin-mediated brain-heart interactions. Cardiol J 2014;21(3):220–8.

34. Frustaci A, Loperfido F, Gentiloni N, et al. Catecholamine-induced cardiomyopathy in multiple endocrine neoplasia: a histologic, ultrastructural, and biochemical study. Chest 1991;99(2):382–5.

35. Samuels MA. The brain-heart connection. Circulation 2007;116(1):77–84.

36. Kastaun S, Schwarz NP, Juenemann M, et al. Cortisol awakening and stress response, personality and psychiatric profiles in patients with takotsubo cardiomyopathy. Heart 2014;100(22):1786–92.

37. Roberts AD, Wessely S, Chalder T. Salivary cortisol response to awakening in chronic fatigue syndrome. Br J Psychiatry 2004;184(2):136–41.

38. Riva R, Mork PJ, Westgaard RH, et al. Comparison of the cortisol awakening response in women with shoulder and neck pain and women with fibromyalgia. Psychoneuroendocrinology 2012;37(2): 299–306.

39. Rohleder N, Joksimovic L, Wolf JM, et al. Hypocortisolism and increased glucocorticoid sensitivity of pro-inflammatory cytokine production in Bosnian war refugees with posttraumatic stress disorder. Biol Psychiatry 2004;55(7):745–51.

40. Hellhammer DH, Wade S. Endocrine correlates of stress vulnerability. Psychother Psychosom 1993; 60:8–17.

41. Kvetnansky R, Fukuhara K, Pacak K. Endogenous glucocorticoids restrain catecholamine synthesis and release at rest and during immobilization stress in rats. Endocrinology 1993;133:1411–9.

42. Golczynska A, Lenders JW, Goldstein DS. Glucocorticoid-induced sympathoinhibition in humans. Clin Pharmacol Ther 1995;58(1):90–8.

43. Het S, Schoofs D, Rohleder N, et al. Stress-induced cortisol level elevations are associated with reduced negative affect after stress: indications for a mood-buffering cortisol effect. Psychosom Med 2012; 74(1):23–32.

44. Mendelsohn ME, Karas RH. The protective effects of estrogen on the cardiovascular system. N Engl J Med 1999;340(23):1801–11.

45. Vitale C, Mendelsohn ME, Rosano GM. Gender differences in the cardiovascular effect of sex hormones. Nat Rev Cardiol 2009;6(8):532–42.

46. Kaski JC, Cox ID, Crook JR, et al. Differential plasma endothelin levels in subgroups of patients with angina and angiographically normal coronary arteries. Coronary Artery Disease Research Group. Am Heart J 1998;136(3):412–7.

47. Martin EA, Prasad A, Rihal CS, et al. Endothelial function and vascular response to mental stress are impaired in patients with apical ballooning syndrome. J Am Coll Cardiol 2010;56(22):1840–6.

48. Ueyama T, Kasamatsu K, Hano T, et al. Catecholamines and estrogen are involved in the pathogenesis of emotional stress-induced acute heart attack. Ann N Y Acad Sci 2008;1148:479–85.

49. Ueyama T, Ishikura F, Matsuda A, et al. Chronic estrogen supplementation following ovariectomy improves the emotional stress-induced cardiovascular responses by indirect action on the nervous system and by direct action on the heart. Circ J 2007;71(4): 565–73.

50. Cao X, Zhou C, Chong J, et al. Estrogen resisted stress-induced cardiomyopathy through increasing the activity of β_2AR-Gαs signal pathway in female rats. Int J Cardiol 2015;187(1):377–86.

51. Grohe C, Kahlert S, Lobbert K, et al. Cardiac myocytes and fibroblasts contain functional estrogen receptors. FEBS Lett 1997;416(1):107–12.

52. Bupha-Intr T, Wattanapermpool J. Regulatory role of ovarian sex hormones in calcium uptake activity of cardiac sarcoplasmic reticulum. Am J Physiol Heart Circ Physiol 2006;291(3):H1101–8.

53. Wright PT, Tranter MH, Morley-Smith AC, et al. Pathophysiology of Takotsubo syndrome. Circ J 2014; 78(7):1550–8.

54. Nef HM, Möllmann H, Troidl C, et al. Abnormalities in intracellular Ca2+ regulation contribute to the path-omechanism of Tako-Tsubo cardiomyopathy. Eur Heart J 2009;30(17):2155–64.

55. Nef HM, Möllmann H, Hilpert P, et al. Activated cell survival cascade protects cardiomyocytes from cell death in Tako-Tsubo cardiomyopathy. Eur J Heart Fail 2009;11(8):758–64.

56. Nef HM, Möllmann H, Troidl C, et al. Expression profiling of cardiac genes in Tako-Tsubo cardiomy-opathy: insight into a new cardiac entity. J Mol Cell Cardiol 2008;44(2):395–404.

57. Pison L, De Vusser P, Mullens W. Apical ballooning in relatives. Heart 2004;90(12):e67.

58. Cherian J, Angelis D, Filiberti A, et al. Can takotsubo cardiomyopathy be familial? Int J Cardiol 2007; 121(1):74–5.

59. Kumar G, Holmes DR, Prasad A. "Familial" apical ballooning syndrome (Takotsubo cardiomyopathy). Int J Cardiol 2010;144(3):444–5.

60. Zaroff JG, Pawlikowska L, Miss JC, et al. Adreno-ceptor polymorphisms and the risk of cardiac injury and dysfunction after subarachnoid hemorrhage. Stroke 2006;37(7):1680–5.

61. Sharkey SW, Maron BJ, Nelson P, et al. Adrenergic receptor polymorphisms in patients with stress (tako-tsubo) cardiomyopathy. J Cardiol 2009; 53(1):53–7.

62. Vriz O, Minisini R, Citro R, et al. Analysis of beta1 and beta2-adrenergic receptors polymorphism in patients with apical ballooning cardiomyopathy. Acta Cardiol 2011;66(6):787–90.

63. Spinelli L, Trimarco V, Di Marino S, et al. L41Q polymorphism of the G protein coupled receptor kinase 5 is associated with left ventricular apical ballooning syndrome. Eur J Heart Fail 2010;12(1):13–6.

64. Goodloe AH, Evans JM, Middha S, et al. Character-izing genetic variation of adrenergic signalling path-ways in Takotsubo (stress) cardiomyopathy exomes. Eur J Heart Fail 2014;16(9):942–9.

65. Summers MR, Lennon RJ, Prasad A. Pre-morbid psychiatric and cardiovascular diseases in apical ballooning syndrome (tako-tsubo/stress-induced cardiomyopathy). Potential pre-disposing factors? J Am Coll Cardiol 2010;55(7): 700–1.

66. Delmas C, Lairez O, Mulin E, et al. Anxiodepressive disorders and chronic psychological stress are associated with Tako-Tsubo cardiomyopathy - new physiopathological hypothesis. Circ J 2013;77(1): 175–80.

67. Scantlebury DC, Prasad A, Rabinstein AA, et al. Prevalence of migraine and Raynaud phenomenon in women with apical ballooning syndrome (takot-subo or stress cardiomyopathy). Am J Cardiol 2013;111(9):1284–8.

68. Cao M, Zhang S, Wang K, et al. Personality traits in migraine and tension-type headaches: a five-factor model study. Psychopathology 2002;35(4): 254–8.

69. Ishii M, Shimizu S, Sakairi Y, et al. MAOA, MTHFR, and TNF-β genes polymorphisms and personality traits in the pathogenesis of migraine. Mol Cell Bio-chem 2012;363(1–2):357–66.

70. Scantlebury DC, Rohe DE, Best PJ, et al. Stress-coping skills and neuroticism in apical ballooning syndrome (takotsubo/stress cardiomyopathy). Open Heart 2016;3(1):e000312.

71. Compare A, Bigi R, Orrego PS, et al. Type D person-ality is associated with the development of stress cardiomyopathy following emotional triggers. Ann Behav Med 2013;45(3):299–307.

72. Del Pace S, Parodi G, Bellandi B, et al. Anxiety trait in patients with stress-induced cardiomyopathy: a case-control study. Clin Res Cardiol 2011;100(6):523–9.

73. Ito K, Sugihara H, Katoh S, et al. Assessment of ta-kotsubo (ampulla) cardiomyopathy using 99mTc-te-trofosmin myocardial SPECT–comparison with acute coronary syndrome. Ann Nucl Med 2003; 17(2):115–22.

74. Kurisu S, Sato H, Kawagoe T, et al. Tako-tsubo-like left ventricular dysfunction with ST-segment eleva-tion: a novel cardiac syndrome mimicking acute myocardial infarction. Am Heart J 2002;143(3): 448–55.

75. Elesber A, Lerman A, Bybee KA, et al. Myocar-dial perfusion in apical ballooning syndrome correlate of myocardial injury. Am Heart J 2006; 152(3):469.e9-13.

76. Kume T, Akasaka T, Kawamoto T, et al. Assessment of coronary microcirculation in patients with takotsubo-like left ventricular dysfunction. Circ J 2005;69(8):934–9.

77. Rigo F, Sicari R, Citro R, et al. Diffuse, marked, reversible impairment in coronary microcirculation in stress cardiomyopathy: a Doppler transthoracic echo study. Ann Med 2009;41(6):462–70.

78. Cimarelli S, Sauer F, Morel O, et al. Transient left ven-tricular dysfunction syndrome: patho-physiological bases through nuclear medicine imaging. Int J Car-diol 2010;144(2):212–8.

79. Ito K, Sugihara H, Kawasaki T, et al. Assessment of ampulla (Takotsubo) cardiomyopathy with coronary angiography, two-dimensional echocardiography and 99mTc-tetrofosmin myocardial single photon emission computed tomography. Ann Nucl Med 2001;15(4):351–5.

80. Kurisu S, Inoue I, Kawagoe T, et al. Myocardial perfusion and fatty acid metabolism in patients with tako-tsubo-like left ventricular dysfunction. J Am Coll Cardiol 2003;41(5):743–8.

81. Yoshida T, Hibino T, Kako N, et al. A pathophysio-logic study of tako-tsubo cardiomyopathy with

F-18 fluorodeoxyglucose positron emission tomography. Eur Heart J 2007;28(21):2598–604.

82. Murry CE, Jennings RB, Reimer KA. Preconditioning with ischemia: a delay of lethal cell injury in ischemic myocardium. Circulation 1986;74(5): 1124–36.

83. Redfors B, Shao Y, Oldfors A, et al. Normal apical myocardial perfusion in the rat model with Takotsubo syndrome: is subsequent microvascular dysfunction and hypoperfusion an epiphenomenon? Reply. Eur Heart J Cardiovasc Imaging 2014;15(1):110–1.

84. Redfors B, Shao Y, Ali A, et al. Are ischemic stunning, conditioning, and "takotsubo" different sides to the same coin? Int J Cardiol 2014;172(2):490–1.

85. Patel SM, Lerman A, Lennon RJ, et al. Impaired coronary microvascular reactivity in women with apical ballooning syndrome (Takotsubo/stress cardiomyopathy). Eur Heart J Acute Cardiovasc Care 2013; 2:147–52.

86. Dib C, Asirvatham S, Elesber A, et al. Clinical correlates and prognostic significance of electrocardiographic abnormalities in apical ballooning syndrome (Takotsubo/stress-induced cardiomyopathy). Am Heart J 2009;157(5):933–8.

87. Jaguszewski M, Osipova J, Ghadri JR, et al. A signature of circulating microRNAs differentiates takotsubo cardiomyopathy from acute myocardial infarction. Eur Heart J 2014;35(15):999–1006.

88. Ibanez B, Navarro F, Cordoba M, et al. Tako-tsubo transient left ventricular apical ballooning: is intravascular ultrasound the key to resolve the enigma? Heart 2005;91(1):102–4.

89. Haghi D, Roehm S, Hamm K, et al. Takotsubo cardiomyopathy is not due to plaque rupture: an intravascular ultrasound study. Clin Cardiol 2010;33(5): 307–10.

90. Hoyt J, Lerman A, Lennon RJ, et al. Left anterior descending artery length and coronary atherosclerosis in apical ballooning syndrome (Takotsubo/stress induced cardiomyopathy). Int J Cardiol 2010; 145(1):112–5.

91. El Mahmoud R, Mansencal N, Pilliere R, et al. Prevalence and characteristics of left ventricular outflow tract obstruction in Tako-Tsubo syndrome. Am Heart J 2008;156(3):543–8.

92. Merli E, Sutcliffe S, Gori M, et al. Tako-Tsubo cardiomyopathy: new insights into the possible underlying pathophysiology. Eur J Echocardiogr 2006;7(1):53–61.

93. Alter P, Figiel JH, Rominger MB. Increased ventricular wall stress and late gadolinium enhancement in Takotsubo cardiomyopathy. Int J Cardiol 2014; 172(1):e184–6.

94. Schultz T, Shao Y, Redfors B, et al. Stress-induced cardiomyopathy in Sweden: evidence for different ethnic predisposition and altered cardio-circulatory status. Cardiology 2012;122(3):180–6.

95. Redfors B, Ali A, Shao Y, et al. Different catecholamines induce different patterns of takotsubo-like cardiac dysfunction in an apparently afterload dependent manner. Int J Cardiol 2014;174(2): 330–6.

The Sympathetic Nervous System in the Pathogenesis of Takotsubo Syndrome

Ilan S. Wittstein, MD

KEYWORDS

- Takotsubo syndrome • Stress cardiomyopathy • Sympathetic nervous system • Catecholamines
- Ventricular ballooning

KEY POINTS

- Enhanced sympathetic stimulation seems to be central to the pathogenesis of takotsubo syndrome.
- Catecholamines may affect cardiac function in takotsubo syndrome through a variety of mechanisms, including epicardial spasm, microvascular dysfunction, and direct myocyte injury from adrenergic-receptor–mediated calcium overload.
- Risk factors that increase sympathetic tone and/or enhance myocyte and microvascular catecholamine sensitivity may increase individual susceptibility to takotsubo syndrome.

INTRODUCTION

There is considerable evidence supporting a strong association between acute psychological stress and cardiovascular morbidity and mortality. Case-crossover studies have demonstrated that the risk of myocardial infarction more than doubles following acute emotional triggers, such as anger and sadness[1,2]; large population-based studies have shown that emotionally charged events, such as earthquakes,[3] acts of terrorism,[4] and even sporting events,[5] are associated with an increased risk of myocardial infarction and ventricular arrhythmia. More recently, it has become increasingly clear that acute psychological stress can also have a direct effect on cardiac contractile function; during the past 15 years, a novel syndrome of acute systolic heart failure precipitated by emotional or physical stress has been reported. The clinical features of *takotsubo*

syndrome (TS), also referred to as stress cardiomyopathy, left ventricular apical ballooning syndrome, and broken heart syndrome, have been well described in the medical literature[6–8] and are reviewed in subsequent articles of this issue. Despite the increased awareness of TS by clinicians worldwide, the precise pathophysiology of this unique syndrome remains elusive and poorly understood. Numerous mechanisms have been proposed, but the preponderance of evidence suggests that the contractile dysfunction characteristic of TS is likely catecholamine mediated.[9] Increased sympathetic stimulation may induce transient myocardial stunning through a variety of mechanisms that include epicardial spasm, ischemia due to microvascular dysfunction, and direct cardiomyocyte toxicity from catecholamine-mediated calcium overload. This article summarizes the evidence supporting enhanced sympathetic stimulation as central to

Disclosure: The author has nothing to disclose.
Division of Cardiology, The Johns Hopkins University School of Medicine, 7125 Zayed Tower, 1800 Orleans Street, Baltimore, MD 21287, USA
E-mail address: iwittste@jhmi.edu

Heart Failure Clin 12 (2016) 485–498
http://dx.doi.org/10.1016/j.hfc.2016.06.012
1551-7136/16/$ – see front matter

the pathogenesis of TS. Further, risk factors are reviewed that may influence individual susceptibility to TS by increasing sympathetic tone and/or by augmenting myocyte and microvascular catecholamine sensitivity.

A PARADIGM FOR SYMPATHETIC STIMULATION AND TAKOTSUBO SYNDROME

Fig. 1 illustrates a proposed paradigm for how sympathetic stimulation may be implicated in the development of TS. First, an individual is exposed to an acute stressor, which may be either emotional or physical. The physiologic response that follows is activation of the sympathetic nervous system (SNS) and release of catecholamines. Depending on the specific nature of the acute trigger, the predominant sympathetic response may be either sympathoneural resulting in local myocardial norepinephrine release or adrenomedullary hormonal leading to an increase in blood born catecholamines. This catecholamine surge may then affect the heart through a variety of pathophysiologic mechanisms, including epicardial spasm, microvascular dysfunction, and direct cardiomyocyte injury. Individual susceptibility to developing clinical TS is determined in large part by a variety of factors that may amplify the sympathetic response and/or enhance myocyte and microvascular sensitivity to catecholamines.

Some of these risk factors that have been suggested from clinical observations and basic research are discussed in more detail later in this article.

EVIDENCE SUPPORTING THE CENTRAL ROLE OF SYMPATHETIC NERVOUS SYSTEM ACTIVATION IN TAKOTSUBO SYNDROME
Presence of an Acute Trigger

In most patients presenting with TS, an antecedent acute emotional or physical stressor can be identified. The observation of this temporal relationship is precisely what led investigators to initially suspect a sympathetic pathogenesis and to refer to the syndrome as *stress cardiomyopathy*.[6] Early reports highlighted primarily the emotional triggers of TS, but increased recognition of the syndrome has made it clear that TS can also be precipitated by a wide variety of physical stressors.[10] Many investigators initially thought that a dramatic stressor and subsequent massive catecholamine surge were required to precipitate TS. It is now clear, however, that even minor stressors can trigger the syndrome and that roughly 30% of patients with TS have no identifiable trigger at all.[11,12] The absence of an identifiable dramatic stressor, however, does not exclude a sympathetically mediated pathogenesis. As is suggested later in this article, even a relatively mild stressor

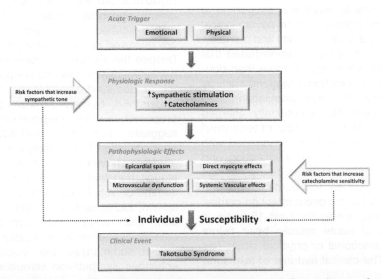

Fig. 1. A proposed paradigm illustrating the link between acute stress and the syndrome of stress cardiomyopathy. Acute emotional or physical stress results in activation of the sympathetic nervous system and an increase in local myocardial catecholamine levels. Catecholamines may mediate myocardial stunning through a variety of mechanisms that include coronary vasospasm, microvascular dysfunction, and myocyte calcium overload. Risk factors that enhance sympathetic tone and/or myocardial sensitivity to catecholamines likely increase individual susceptibility to takotsubo syndrome during periods of acute stress. (*Adapted from* Bhattacharyya MR, Steptoe A. Emotional triggers of acute coronary syndromes: strength of evidence, biological processes, and clinical implications. Prog Cardiovasc Dis 2007;49:354.)

may be sufficient to precipitate TS in particularly vulnerable individuals who may have either increased sympathetic tone at baseline or enhanced myocyte or microvascular catecholamine sensitivity.

Association with High Catecholamine States

TS has been observed in several clinical conditions known to be associated with exaggerated SNS activity. Numerous investigators have reported both apical and nonapical variants of TS in the setting of pheochromocytoma or functional paraganglioma.[13–15] In one systematic literature review, pheochromocytoma occurred in 13% of the reported cases of TS.[13] Coupez and colleagues[16] found that the incidence of catecholaminergic tumors in their cohort of patients with TS was 7.5%, an incidence significantly higher than what has been reported in the general population. TS has also been associated with a wide variety of central neurologic insults that are known to result in hyperadrenergic stimulation, such as subarachnoid hemorrhage, ischemic or hemorrhagic stroke, seizure, encephalitis, traumatic brain injury, acute hydrocephalus, posterior reversible encephalopathy syndrome, and even severe headache.[17–21] Patients with stroke at or near the insular cortex with resulting overflow of sympathetic nerve trafficking seem to be particularly susceptible to TS.[22] TS has also been reported with several other conditions of enhanced sympathetic tone, including postural orthostatic tachycardia syndrome,[23] alcohol and opioid withdrawal,[24,25] and cocaine use.[26]

Administration of Exogenous Catecholamines

Numerous investigators have reported that TS can be precipitated by the acute administration of catecholamines and beta agonists. Abraham and colleagues[27] demonstrated that all 3 ventricular ballooning variants could result not only from supratherapeutic doses of epinephrine during procedures but also from standard doses of dobutamine typically used in clinical practice. TS has also been reported following the use of an EpiPen (Mylan, Canonsburg, PA) for an allergic reaction[28] as well as following the ingestion of amphetamines[29] and pseudoephedrine.[30] These observations reinforce the idea that sympathetic stimulation is central to the pathogenesis of TS and that the syndrome may be mediated in some cases through blood-born catecholamines and sympathomimetics.

Clinical Features

Electrocardiogram

The unique electrocardiographic (ECG) findings seen in TS have been well described.[6,31,32] Although there is no pathognomonic ECG in TS, characteristic findings include ST-segment elevation at the time of presentation in about half of the cases, deep and diffuse T-wave inversion, and a markedly prolonged QT interval (**Fig. 2**A). These ECG findings occur in the absence of obstructive coronary disease in most cases of TS and are strikingly similar to the changes observed following acute central neurologic injury that were described more than half a century ago.[33] Catecholamines are known to increase the QT interval,[34,35] and experimental animal models

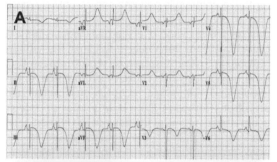

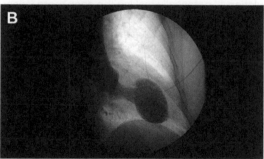

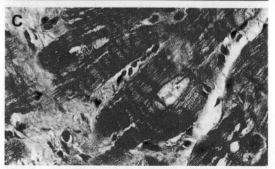

Fig. 2. Some of the classic clinical features observed during the acute phase of TS. All are thought to be catecholamine mediated and include deep diffuse T-wave inversion and prolonged QT interval on ECG (A), left ventricular apical ballooning seen with ventriculography (B), and a mononuclear lymphocytic infiltrate with contraction band necrosis on endomyocardial biopsy (C).

have demonstrated that these characteristic ECG findings can be reproduced through stimulation of the central SNS and attenuated by transection of the cervical spinal cord.[36] These observations support the idea that the ECG abnormalities in TS are secondary to sympathetic disruption and local myocardial catecholamine release and not primarily the result of cardiac ischemia.

Ventricular ballooning

Perhaps the most defining characteristic of TS is the unusual left ventricular contractile pattern observed at the time of presentation. Several ballooning variants have been previously described,[8,37,38] and all are characterized by wall motion abnormalities that extend beyond a single vascular territory (see Fig. 2B). An ischemic cause for these contractile patterns seems unlikely given that multiple vascular distributions are affected despite the absence of epicardial disease in most patients. It has been suggested that the various ballooning patterns observed in TS may reflect local myocardial differences in sympathetic innervation and adrenergic receptor distribution and sensitivity. Although there is a greater density of sympathetic nerves at the base of the human heart than in the apex,[39] the beta-receptors in the apex may be more responsive to sympathetic stimulation,[40] potentially making the apex more vulnerable to sudden catecholamine surges. Lyon and colleagues[41] have suggested that the apical contractile dysfunction in TS results from an epinephrine-mediated switch from G_s to G_i protein signaling via the β_2-adrenergic receptor, though this mechanism does not readily explain the patterns observed in the nonapical ballooning variants. Bonnemeier and colleagues[42] have demonstrated that the apical ballooning variant may result from activation of the left stellate ganglion and cardiac sympathetic nerves, whereas the midventricular variant may occur following activation of the right stellate ganglion and cardiac sympathetic nerves. Although the precise mechanism remains unclear, it seems likely that the wall motion abnormalities in TS result from disruption of the cardiac neural supply system and that involvement of different branches of the cardiac sympathetic system leads to the various ballooning patterns.

Histopathology

Histopathologic findings in patients with TS also seem to support a sympathetic pathogenesis. Endomyocardial biopsy specimens have demonstrated contraction band necrosis and an interstitial mononuclear inflammatory response that differs from the polymorphonuclear inflammation typically seen with infarction (see Fig. 2C).[6,43]

Contraction band necrosis is a unique form of myocyte injury characterized by hypercontracted sarcomeres and dense eosinophilic bands. It has been described in high catecholamine states, such as pheochromocytoma,[44] subarachnoid hemorrhage,[45] and violent assault[46]; its presence in patients with TS reinforces that catecholamines may be an important link between acute stress and cardiac injury. This idea is also suggested by the observations at autopsy of not only contraction band necrosis but also a massive expression of β_1 adrenergic receptors in the subendocardial and deep myocardial layers of patients who died of TS.[47]

Assessment of Sympathetic Tone in Takotsubo Syndrome

Several methods have been used to assess sympathetic tone in TS. Although the data have at times been inconsistent, the preponderance of evidence suggests that SNS activity is enhanced during the acute phase of the syndrome.

Plasma catecholamines

Measurement of plasma catecholamines in patients with TS has yielded variable results. In patients with TS due to emotional triggers, Wittstein and colleagues[6] demonstrated massively elevated plasma catecholamines and stress-related neuropeptides compared with patients with Killip III myocardial infarction. Similar plasma catecholamine levels have been reported in patients with TS due to pheochromocytoma.[14] Elevated coronary sinus norepinephrine levels have also been detected in patients with TS, suggesting an increase in local myocardial catecholamine release.[48] In contrast, Y-Hassan and Henareh[49] found only mild to moderate elevation of plasma norepinephrine in 48% of patients with TS presenting with both emotional and physical triggers. Similarly, Madhavan and colleagues[50] saw no elevation in plasma or urinary metanephrines in a series of patients with TS presenting mostly with physical stressors. Reasons for these inconsistent findings likely include the heterogeneity of stressors between studies, the timing of the blood draw in relation to the initial trigger, and differences in technique between laboratories. The absence of elevated plasma catecholamines, however, does not rule out a sympathetic mechanism of TS. It is possible that elevated plasma levels might only be detected in individuals with primarily adrenomedullary hormonal activation and would not necessarily be expected to correlate with an increase in local myocardial catecholamines due to enhanced sympathoneural stimulation.

Heart rate variability

Several investigators have performed heart rate variability (HRV) analysis in both the acute and follow-up phases of TS.[51,52] Both frequency and time-domain parameters of HRV have demonstrated sympathetic predominance and depression of cardiac parasympathetic activity at the time of presentation, followed by recovery of sympathovagal balance by 3 months (**Fig. 3**).

Microneurography

Investigators have used microneurography to measure muscle sympathetic nerve activity (MSNA) in patients with TS. MSNA provides a direct and dynamic assessment of postganglionic SNS activity. Vaccaro and colleagues[53] found that patients with TS had significantly increased MSNA compared with a control group with acute decompensated heart failure (**Fig. 4**). All of the subjects in this study underwent microneurography within 72 hours of symptom onset. In contrast, Sverrisdottir and colleagues[54] found that patients with TC had a decrease in MSNA compared with healthy matched controls. This latter study provides less information regarding sympathetic tone during the acute phase of TS because more than half of the subjects were studied in the recovery phase at 1 to 6 months.

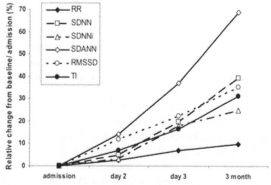

Fig. 3. Relative changes in indices of heart rate variability in patients presenting with TS. Suppression of these indices suggests sympathetic predominance at the time of admission, with gradual recovery of cardiac autonomic tone over a 3-month period. RMSSD, root mean square of consecutive difference of normal-to-normal intervals; RR, RR interval; SDANN, standard deviation of the averages of normal-to-normal intervals for all 5-minute segments; SDNN, standard deviation of normal-to-normal intervals; SDNNi, mean standard deviation of normal-to-normal-intervals for 5 minute segments; TI, geometric triangular index. (*From* Ortak J, Khattab K, Barantke M, et al. Evolution of cardiac autonomic nervous activity indices in patients presenting with transient left ventricular apical ballooning. Pacing Clin Electrophysiol 2009;32:S24; with permission.)

Baroreflex function

Only one group has attempted to assess baroreflex function during the acute phase of TS. Using microneurography, spontaneous baroreflex control of sympathetic activity was determined by the slope of the regression line representing the relationship between spontaneous diastolic blood pressure and MSNA.[53] Compared with subjects with decompensated heart failure, subjects with TS had a significant decrease in spontaneous baroreflex control of sympathetic activity, providing more evidence that sympathetic dysregulation may be central to the pathophysiology of TS.

Cardiac imaging

Myocardial scintigraphy using the norepinephrine analogue ^{123}I-metaiodobenzyl-guanidine (MIBG) has been used to study cardiac sympathetic innervation in patients with TS. Several studies have demonstrated a decreased heart/mediastinum ratio and an increased washout rate during the acute phase of TS suggesting abnormalities in presynaptic norepinephrine uptake and an increase in presynaptic catecholamine release.[55–57] Areas of decreased ^{123}I-MIBG uptake frequently coincide with focal areas of hypokinesis or akinesis during the acute phase of TS, and myocardial sympathetic function can remain abnormal for several months after ventricular systolic function has fully recovered.[55,58] Enhanced myocardial sympathetic activity during the acute phase of TS has also been demonstrated with PET imaging of the norepinephrine analogue ^{11}C hydroxyephedrine (HED). Decreased ^{11}C-HED in segments of the heart with contractile dysfunction results from increased release from presynaptic neurons and possibly also from impaired neuronal reuptake due to transient dysfunction of the uptake-1 mechanism.[59]

Animal Models of Takotsubo Syndrome

Several animal models have highlighted the central role of the SNS in the pathogenesis of TS. Ueyama and colleagues[60] used immobilization stress to induce left ventricular apical ballooning in rats, and this effect was prevented by pretreating with α and β adrenergic receptor blockers. Similarly, intravenous epinephrine infusion in monkeys resulted in left ventricular apical hypokinesis and myocytolysis, both of which could be attenuated by pretreating with metoprolol.[61] Paur and colleagues[62] demonstrated in a rat model that boluses of epinephrine, but not norepinephrine, produced apical dysfunction and basal hypercontractility characteristic of TS. They demonstrated an apex to base gradient of β_2 receptors and found that apical contractile dysfunction was enhanced with beta-blockers that activate the β_2 adrenergic receptor inhibitory

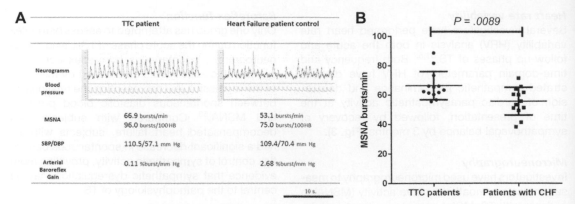

Fig. 4. Microneurographic recording of MSNA in patients with TS compared with patients with acute decompensated heart failure. (*A*) Increased frequency of sympathetic bursts in one patient with TS compared with a control with acute heart failure. (*B*) Comparison of mean MSNA, expressed in burst per minute, between a group of patients with TS and a control group with acute decompensated heart failure. CHF, congestive hear failure; DBP, diastolic blood pressure; HB, heart beats; SBP, systolic blood pressure; TTC, takotsubo cardiomyopathy. (*From* Vaccaro A, Despas F, Delmas C, et al. Direct evidences for sympathetic hyperactivity and baroreflex impairment in tako tsubo cardiomyopathy. PLoS One 2014;9:e93278; with permission.)

G-protein (β_2AR-G_i) pathway, whereas inactivation of G_i with pertussis toxin decreased cardiac dysfunction and increased mortality. The investigators hypothesized that selective apical dysfunction likely resulted from biased agonism of epinephrine for the β_2 adrenergic receptor stimulatory G-protein (β_2AR-Gs) at low concentrations and β_2AR-G_i at high concentrations, a strategy that may have evolved to minimize catecholamine-mediated cardiotoxicity during periods of acute stress. Shao and colleagues were able to reproduce TS in rats with the β-adrenergic agonist isoprenaline and found a higher intracellular lipid content in the akinetic segments. β_2 adrenergic receptor blockade or G_i pathway inhibition decreased akinesis and lipid accumulation but significantly increased acute mortality, once again highlighting the potential protective mechanism of transient catecholamine myocardial depression.[63] More recently, however, Redfors and colleagues[64] were able to induce TS in rats with intraperitoneal injection of several different catecholamines. Using real-time echocardiographic and hemodynamic monitoring, they concluded that catecholamine-mediated TS was afterload dependent and did not depend on stimulation of specific adrenergic receptor subtypes.

PATHOPHYSIOLOGIC EFFECTS OF INCREASED SYMPATHETIC STIMULATION IN TAKOTSUBO SYNDROME

The precise mechanism in which exaggerated sympathetic stimulation induces TS remains uncertain. Several potential pathophysiologic mechanisms have been proposed and are briefly reviewed (see **Fig. 1**).

Plaque Rupture

Catecholamine-mediated plaque rupture was one of the earliest proposed mechanisms to explain TS. Some investigators argued that apical ballooning likely resulted from plaque rupture and transient coronary thrombosis in a large wrap-around left anterior descending (LAD) coronary artery.[65] Although eccentric atherosclerotic plaque in the mid LAD has been reported in a small number of patients with TS, most studies using intravascular ultrasound have failed to detect plaque.[66,67] It is also now clear that apical ballooning can occur in the absence of a wrap-around LAD and that this anatomy is no more prevalent in TS than in a control population.[68] Further, ischemia from a wrap-around LAD would not explain the nonapical ballooning variants that have been well described. All of these observations support the conclusion that catecholamine-mediated plaque rupture with aborted myocardial infarction is not the primary pathophysiologic mechanism responsible for TS.

Coronary Vasoconstriction

It has been proposed that acute endothelial dysfunction due to sudden adrenergic stimulation could cause multivessel coronary spasm, transient ischemia, and myocardial contractile dysfunction in multiple vascular territories. Angelini[69] demonstrated severe multivessel coronary spasm with the intracoronary administration of acetylcholine[69] and suggested that the variant of left ventricular ballooning observed in patients with TS may depend on the specific coronary branches affected.[70] Although coronary spasm may play a role in some patients with TS, most patients have no evidence of epicardial spasm at the time of angiography, even when provocative agents are used.[71] Even in Japan where the incidence of coronary vasospasm is particularly high, acetylcholine infusion was only able to provoke epicardial spasm in approximately 20% of patients with TS.[8] These observations suggest that, although abnormal coronary vasomotion may play a pathogenic role in a subset of patients with TS, sympathetically mediated epicardial spasm is unlikely the primary mechanism of myocardial stunning in most patients with this syndrome.

Microvascular Dysfunction

Sympathetically mediated microvascular dysfunction is another proposed pathophysiologic mechanism of TS. Decreased coronary flow reserve (CFR) has been demonstrated noninvasively during the acute phase of TS with PET/computed tomography[72] and with echocardiography following the infusion of adenosine[73] and dipyridamole.[74] Decreased CFR has also been demonstrated invasively using Doppler flow wires,[75] and patients with TS who undergo angiography have elevated thrombolysis in myocardial infarction (TIMI) frame counts in all 3 epicardial vessels[76] as well as abnormal TIMI myocardial perfusion grades in multiple vascular territories,[77] findings that suggest a diffuse microcirculatory process. In an endomyocardial biopsy study of TS, Uchida[78] found elevated catecholamine levels and evidence of microvascular endothelial cell apoptosis, supporting the idea that sympathetically mediated microvascular injury could be pathogenic during the acute phase of the syndrome. Further evidence suggests that microvascular dysfunction in TS may be a systemic process that involves more than just the coronary microcirculation. During the acute phase, patients with TS have marked impairment in brachial artery flow–mediated dilation compared with patients with myocardial infarction and with healthy controls; this abnormality gradually improves over several weeks.[79]

Direct Myocyte Effects

Transient left ventricular dysfunction in TS could alternatively result from the direct effects of catecholamines on cardiac myocytes. Catecholamines can decrease myocyte viability through cyclic adenosine monophosphate–mediated calcium overload.[80] Endomyocardial biopsy samples from patients with TS have demonstrated contraction band necrosis, a unique form of myocyte injury that has been associated with states of catecholamine excess.[6] Patients presenting acutely with TS seem to have downregulation of sarcoplasmic Ca^{2+} ATPase (SERCA2a) gene expression, increased expression of sarcolipin, and dephosphorylation of phospholamban, findings that might explain myocardial contractile dysfunction due to decreased calcium affinity.[81] As reviewed earlier, animal models have suggested that high levels of epinephrine may be negatively inotropic due to stimulus trafficking, a proposed mechanism involving a molecular switch of the β_2 adrenergic receptor from the positively inotropic Gs secondary messenger pathway to the negatively inotropic G_i pathway.[41] This switch to G_i signaling may be protective in the acute phase of TS by activating several pathways that reduce catecholamine toxicity and decrease apoptosis.[82,83]

Systemic Vascular Effects

The systemic vascular response to catecholamines may have pathogenic importance in TS through its effect on ventricular-arterial coupling. Acute sympathetic stimulation may result in systemic vasoconstriction, increased ventricular intracavitary pressure, increased wall stress, and regional contractile dysfunction. A recent animal model demonstrated the importance of increased afterload in the development of TS and the particular ballooning variant observed.[64] It has been observed, however, that some patients with TS develop paradoxically low peripheral vascular resistance, possibly secondary to vasodilatory catecholamines and oxidative stress in the peripheral vasculature.[84] The sympathetic regulation of systemic vascular tone in response to acute stress seems to be a dynamic process during the early phase of TS and may be important in determining both phenotype and subsequent clinical course of patients with this condition through its effect on ventricular-arterial coupling.

FACTORS THAT MAY INCREASE SUSCEPTIBILITY TO TAKOTSUBO SYNDROME

Psychological and physical stressors are ubiquitous and a normal part of everyday human life, but only a relatively small number of individuals develop TS, which suggests that there are risk factors that make certain individuals particularly vulnerable. If one accepts the premise that sympathetic stimulation is central to the pathogenesis of TS, then these risk factors likely increase susceptibility by augmenting the sympathetic stress response and/or increasing myocyte and microcirculatory sensitivity to catecholamines.

As mentioned earlier in this article, it was once widely thought that a dramatic trigger and massive catecholamine surge were required to precipitate TS. It is now well recognized that the syndrome can occur in the setting of seemingly mild stressors or no identifiable trigger at all. An explanation for this observation is illustrated in **Fig. 5** and proposes that the amount of sympathetic stimulation needed to precipitate TS may be inversely related to the number of risk factors an individual has that increase sympathetic tone and/or enhance catecholamine sensitivity.

Factors That Increase Sympathetic Tone

Hormonal factors

The striking preponderance of postmenopausal women in all series of TS to date suggests a pathogenic hormonal influence. Female hormones exert important influences on the autonomic nervous system. As women age, there are significant decreases in cardiac vagal tone and baroreflex sensitivity as well as an increase in sympathetic activation.[85] In postmenopausal women, cardiovascular β-adrenoreceptor responsiveness is decreased and α_1-adrenoreceptor responsiveness is increased, and estrogen decreases the sympathetic response to mental stress.[86] Therefore, sympathetic nervous activity replaces parasympathetic activity as the main regulator of the cardiovascular system as women age, thus, making postmenopausal women particularly susceptible to TS during periods of acute stress.

Mood disorders/anxiety

There is a high prevalence of mood disorders and anxiety in patients with TS. In a retrospective case-control study, Summers and colleagues[87] demonstrated that 68% of patients with TS had either anxiety or depression, and the prevalence of these disorders was higher than in patients with myocardial infarction or in healthy controls.[87] In one of the few prospective trials examining psychological disorders in TS, Delmas and colleagues[88] found the incidence of depression and anxiety to be as high as 78%, which was significantly higher than in patients with acute coronary syndromes. Depressed patients have an exaggerated norepinephrine response to emotional stress,[89] and a subset of patients with major depressive disorders have increased spillover and decreased reuptake of norepinephrine.[90] Decreased catecholamine reuptake due to impairment of the norepinephrine transporter has been reported in some patients with panic disorder and anxiety.[91] In addition, antidepressants, such as selective norepinephrine reuptake inhibitors, may facilitate myocardial stunning by increasing local myocardial catecholamine levels.

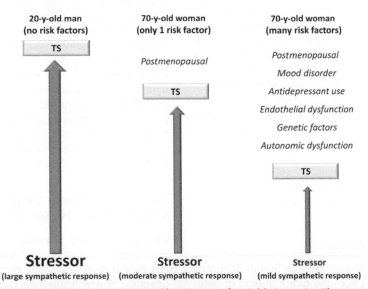

Fig. 5. A model to explain how TS can be precipitated by triggers of variable intensity. The amount of stress needed to precipitate the clinical syndrome depends on individual risk factors that influence catecholamine production and/or myocyte and microvascular sensitivity to sympathetic stimulation. A person with no obvious risk factors (eg, a young man) may require a large catecholamine surge to precipitate TS. In contrast, a person with many risk factors (eg, postmenopausal woman with depression and endothelial dysfunction) may experience the syndrome after just mild sympathetic stimulation due to increased cardiac sensitivity to catecholamines. (*From* Wittstein IS. Stress cardiomyopathy: a syndrome of catecholamine mediated myocardial stunning? Cell Mol Neurobiol 2012;32:855; with permission.)

Medications

Chronic medications that increase basal sympathetic tone may predispose individuals to TS. Dozens of medications with sympathomimetic effects have been associated with an increased risk of developing TS and include antidepressants, β_2 receptor agonists,[92] and decongestants.[30] A comprehensive review of medications associated with TS has been recently presented.[93]

Chronic autonomic dysfunction

There is evidence to suggest that increased sympathetic tone in some patients with TS may be due to baseline autonomic dysfunction. Women with a history of TS demonstrate catecholamine hyperreactivity in response to emotional stress and exercise when compared with healthy controls.[94] Norcliffe-Kaufmann and colleagues[95] studied autonomic function in women who had fully recovered from their episodes of TS. Compared with matched healthy controls, women with a history of TS exhibit exaggerated sympathetic responses to emotional and hemodynamic stressors and suppressed parasympathetic modulation of the heart, even years after the index event.[95] The central autonomic response to autonomic challenges, such as Valsalva and cold exposure, is also altered in individuals with a remote history of TS as assessed by functional MRI.[96] These studies suggest that individuals with a history of TS may have chronic sympathetic/parasympathetic imbalance, thus, rendering them particularly vulnerable to acute sympathetic stimulation.

Factors That Increase Catecholamine Sensitivity

Hormonal factors

Estrogen has an important influence on vasomotor tone through the upregulation of endothelial nitric oxide synthase activity,[97] and there is clinical evidence that estrogen can attenuate catecholamine-mediated vasoconstriction.[98] Low estradiol levels in postmenopausal women increase the risk of focal left ventricular wall motion abnormalities following subarachnoid hemorrhage.[99] In animal models of TS, estrogen supplementation in ovariectomized rats attenuates the negative effect of immobilization stress on left ventricular systolic function[100] and protects the myocardium from catecholamines through activation of the β_2AR-G_s signaling pathway.[101] Therefore, by increasing vascular and cardiomyocyte sensitivity to the effects of catecholamines, estrogen depletion may make older women more susceptible to TS during periods of acute stress.

Inherent endothelial dysfunction

Several studies have demonstrated that patients with TS may have inherent endothelial dysfunction and chronic dysregulation of vasomotor tone. Barletta and colleagues[102] performed cold pressor testing (CPT) on women who were 1 to 3 years out from their episode of TS. In contrast to a matched control group, these subjects developed an increase in catecholamines, apical and midventricular wall motion abnormalities, and no increase in coronary flow with CPT. Martin and colleagues[103] used peripheral arterial tonometry to assess endothelial function in subjects with a remote history of TS subjected to mental stress testing. In contrast to a control group of postmenopausal women, these subjects demonstrated increased catecholamine production, impaired vascular vasodilation, and increased vasoconstriction. Using an intracoronary Doppler flow wire in women who had fully recovered from TS, Patel and colleagues[104] demonstrated evidence of severe microvascular dysfunction with infusion of intracoronary acetylcholine. Further, the greatest amount of microcirculatory impairment was observed in women with recurrent episodes of TS. These studies all suggest that individuals with chronic endothelial and microvascular dysfunction may be particularly susceptible to the effects of sympathetic stimulation during periods of acute stress.

Genetic factors

Studies looking for genetic determinants of abnormal adrenergic signaling in TS have yielded conflicting findings. Vriz and colleagues[105] demonstrated an increased genotype frequency of a beta 1 adrenergic receptor (β_1AR) polymorphism (amino acid position 389) in patients with TS compared with controls, but Sharkey and colleagues[106] were unable to identify an increase in genotype frequency for either the β_1AR polymorphism (amino acid position 389 and 49) or $\alpha2c$ receptor polymorphism (deletion 322–325) in a cohort of patients with TS. Several groups have examined the frequency of the L41Q polymorphism of the G protein coupled receptor kinase 5 (GRK5). The L41 variant of GRK5 enhances β-adrenergic receptor desensitization and decreases the response to sympathetic stimulation. An increased frequency of this polymorphism was observed in patients with TS compared with controls in 2 small studies[107,108]; but no increase in frequency of GRK5, β_1AR, or $\beta2AR$ polymorphisms was detected in a larger cohort of TS.[109] Larger genetic studies are necessary, but these initial reports raise the intriguing possibility that susceptibility to TS may in some individuals be influenced by genetic determinants of adrenergic cell signaling.

SUMMARY

There is now considerable evidence from both human studies and animal models that enhanced sympathetic stimulation is central to the pathogenesis of TS. Several techniques have been used to assess sympathetic tone in individuals presenting with TS, and most of these studies have demonstrated exaggerated SNS activity during the acute phase of the syndrome. Hyperadrenergic stimulation may result in myocardial stunning through several mechanisms that include epicardial spasm, microvascular dysfunction, direct myocyte injury, and systemic vascular effects that modulate ventricular-arterial coupling. Risk factors that enhance sympathetic tone and/or increase cardiac catecholamine sensitivity seem to increase individual susceptibility to TS. Exciting challenges for the future will be to better characterize these risk factors, to determine whether modulation of these risk factors can reduce the deleterious effects of acute stress on cardiac function, and to elucidate the precise cellular and molecular mechanisms of sympathetically mediated myocardial stunning.

REFERENCES

1. Mittleman MA, Maclure M, Sherwood JB, et al. Triggering of acute myocardial infarction onset by episodes of anger. Determinants of Myocardial Infarction Onset Study Investigators. Circulation 1995;92(7):1720–5.
2. Steptoe A, Strike PC, Perkins-Porras L, et al. Acute depressed mood as a trigger of acute coronary syndromes. Biol Psychiatry 2006;60(8):837–42.
3. Leor J, Poole WK, Kloner RA. Sudden cardiac death triggered by an earthquake. N Engl J Med 1996;334(7):413–9.
4. Meisel SR, Kutz I, Dayan KI, et al. Effect of Iraqi missile war on incidence of acute myocardial infarction and sudden death in Israeli civilians. Lancet 1991;338(8768):660–1.
5. Wilbert-Lampen U, Leistner D, Greven S, et al. Cardiovascular events during World Cup soccer. N Engl J Med 2008;358(5):475–83.
6. Wittstein IS, Thiemann DR, Lima JA, et al. Neurohumoral features of myocardial stunning due to sudden emotional stress. N Engl J Med 2005; 352(6):539–48.
7. Sharkey SW, Lesser JR, Zenovich AG, et al. Acute and reversible cardiomyopathy provoked by stress in women from the United States. Circulation 2005; 111(4):472–9.
8. Tsuchihashi K, Ueshima K, Uchida T, et al. Transient left ventricular apical ballooning without coronary artery stenosis: a novel heart syndrome mimicking acute myocardial infarction. Angina Pectoris-Myocardial Infarction Investigations in Japan. J Am Coll Cardiol 2001;38(1):11–8.
9. Wittstein IS. Stress cardiomyopathy: a syndrome of catecholamine-mediated myocardial stunning? Cell Mol Neurobiol 2012;32(5):847–57.
10. Sharkey SW, Windenburg DC, Lesser JR, et al. Natural history and expansive clinical profile of stress (tako-tsubo) cardiomyopathy. J Am Coll Cardiol 2010;55(4):333–41.
11. Pelliccia F, Parodi G, Greco C, et al. Comorbidities frequency in takotsubo syndrome: an international collaborative systematic review including 1109 patients. Am J Med 2015; 128(6)(654):e611–59.
12. Templin C, Ghadri JR, Diekmann J, et al. Clinical features and outcomes of takotsubo (stress) cardiomyopathy. N Engl J Med 2015;373(10): 929–38.
13. Agarwal V, Kant G, Hans N, et al. Takotsubo-like cardiomyopathy in pheochromocytoma. Int J Cardiol 2011;153(3):241–8.
14. Sharkey SW, McAllister N, Dassenko D, et al. Evidence that high catecholamine levels produced by pheochromocytoma may be responsible for tako-tsubo cardiomyopathy. Am J Cardiol 2015; 115(11):1615–8.
15. Giavarini A, Chedid A, Bobrie G, et al. Acute catecholamine cardiomyopathy in patients with phaeochromocytoma or functional paraganglioma. Heart 2013;99(19):1438–44.
16. Coupez E, Eschalier R, Pereira B, et al. A single pathophysiological pathway in takotsubo cardiomyopathy: catecholaminergic stress. Arch Cardiovasc Dis 2014;107(4):245–52.
17. Abd TT, Hayek S, Cheng JW, et al. Incidence and clinical characteristics of takotsubo cardiomyopathy post-aneurysmal subarachnoid hemorrhage. Int J Cardiol 2014;176(3):1362–4.
18. Finsterer J, Wahbi K. CNS disease triggering takotsubo stress cardiomyopathy. Int J Cardiol 2014; 177(2):322–9.
19. Porto I, Della Bona R, Leo A, et al. Stress cardiomyopathy (tako-tsubo) triggered by nervous system diseases: a systematic review of the reported cases. Int J Cardiol 2013;167(6):2441–8.
20. Summers MR, Madhavan M, Chokka RG, et al. Coincidence of apical ballooning syndrome (takotsubo/stress cardiomyopathy) and posterior reversible encephalopathy syndrome: potential common substrate and pathophysiology? J Card Fail 2012;18(2):120–5.
21. Jalan P, Dhakal L, Pandav V, et al. Status migrainosus as a potential stressor leading to takotsubo cardiomyopathy. Cephalalgia 2012;32(15):1140–3.
22. Yoshimura S, Toyoda K, Ohara T, et al. Takotsubo cardiomyopathy in acute ischemic stroke. Ann Neurol 2008;64(5):547–54.

23. Khurana RK. Takotsubo cardiomyopathy in a patient with postural tachycardia syndrome. Clin Auton Res 2008;18(1):43–7.

24. Harris ZM, Alonso A, Kennedy TP. Adrenergic inhibition with dexmedetomidine to treat stress cardiomyopathy during alcohol withdrawal: a case report and literature review. Case Rep Crit Care 2016; 2016:9693653.

25. Sarcon A, Ghadri JR, Wong G, et al. Takotsubo cardiomyopathy associated with opiate withdrawal. QJM 2014;107(4):301–2.

26. Arora S, Alfayoumi F, Srinivasan V. Transient left ventricular apical ballooning after cocaine use: is catecholamine cardiotoxicity the pathologic link? Mayo Clin Proc 2006;81(6):829–32.

27. Abraham J, Mudd JO, Kapur NK, et al. Stress cardiomyopathy after intravenous administration of catecholamines and beta-receptor agonists. J Am Coll Cardiol 2009;53(15):1320–5.

28. Zubrinich CM, Farouque HM, Rochford SE, et al. Tako-tsubo-like cardiomyopathy after EpiPen administration. Intern Med J 2008;38(11):862–5.

29. Fulcher J, Wilcox I. Basal stress cardiomyopathy induced by exogenous catecholamines in younger adults. Int J Cardiol 2013;168(6):e158–60.

30. Zlotnick DM, Helisch A. Recurrent stress cardiomyopathy induced by Sudafed PE. Ann Intern Med 2012;156(2):171–2.

31. Sharkey SW, Lesser JR, Menon M, et al. Spectrum and significance of electrocardiographic patterns, troponin levels, and thrombolysis in myocardial infarction frame count in patients with stress (takotsubo) cardiomyopathy and comparison to those in patients with ST-elevation anterior wall myocardial infarction. Am J Cardiol 2008;101(12):1723–8.

32. Kosuge M, Kimura K. Electrocardiographic findings of takotsubo cardiomyopathy as compared with those of anterior acute myocardial infarction. J Electrocardiol 2014;47(5):684–9.

33. Burch GE, Meyers R, Abildskov JA. A new electrocardiographic pattern observed in cerebrovascular accidents. Circulation 1954;9(5):719–23.

34. Abildskov JA. Adrenergic effects of the QT interval of the electrocardiogram. Am Heart J 1976;92(2): 210–6.

35. Magnano AR, Talathoti N, Hallur R, et al. Sympathomimetic infusion and cardiac repolarization: the normative effects of epinephrine and isoproterenol in healthy subjects. J Cardiovasc Electrophysiol 2006;17(9):983–9.

36. Porter RW, Kamikawa K, Grreenhoot JH. Persistent electrocardiographic abnormalities experimentally induced by stimulation of the brain. Am Heart J 1962;64:815–9.

37. Hurst RT, Askew JW, Reuss CS, et al. Transient midventricular ballooning syndrome: a new variant. J Am Coll Cardiol 2006;48(3):579–83.

38. Reuss CS, Lester SJ, Hurst RT, et al. Isolated left ventricular basal ballooning phenotype of transient cardiomyopathy in young women. Am J Cardiol 2007;99(10):1451–3.

39. Kawano H, Okada R, Yano K. Histological study on the distribution of autonomic nerves in the human heart. Heart Vessels 2003;18(1):32–9.

40. Mori H, Ishikawa S, Kojima S, et al. Increased responsiveness of left ventricular apical myocardium to adrenergic stimuli. Cardiovasc Res 1993; 27(2):192–8.

41. Lyon AR, Rees PS, Prasad S, et al. Stress (takotsubo) cardiomyopathy–a novel pathophysiological hypothesis to explain catecholamine-induced acute myocardial stunning. Nat Clin Pract Cardiovasc Med 2008;5(1):22–9.

42. Bonnemeier H, Demming T, Weidtmann B, et al. Differential heart rate dynamics in transient left ventricular apical and midventricular ballooning. Heart Rhythm 2010;7(12):1825–32.

43. Nef HM, Mollmann H, Kostin S, et al. Tako-tsubo cardiomyopathy: intraindividual structural analysis in the acute phase and after functional recovery. Eur Heart J 2007;28(20):2456–64.

44. Wilkenfeld C, Cohen M, Lansman SL, et al. Heart transplantation for end-stage cardiomyopathy caused by an occult pheochromocytoma. J Heart Lung Transplant 1992;11(2 Pt 1): 363–6.

45. Neil-Dwyer G, Walter P, Cruickshank JM, et al. Effect of propranolol and phentolamine on myocardial necrosis after subarachnoid haemorrhage. Br Med J 1978;2(6143):990–2.

46. Cebelin MS, Hirsch CS. Human stress cardiomyopathy. Myocardial lesions in victims of homicidal assaults without internal injuries. Hum Pathol 1980;11(2):123–32.

47. D'Errico S, Neri M, Nieddu A, et al. Cardiac beta1-adrenoceptor expression in two stress-induced cardiomyopathy-related deaths. Forensic Sci Int 2011;207(1–3):e8–11.

48. Kume T, Kawamoto T, Okura H, et al. Local release of catecholamines from the hearts of patients with tako-tsubo-like left ventricular dysfunction. Circ J 2008;72(1):106–8.

49. Y-Hassan S, Henareh L. Plasma catecholamine levels in patients with takotsubo syndrome: implications for the pathogenesis of the disease. Int J Cardiol 2014;181:35–8.

50. Madhavan M, Borlaug BA, Lerman A, et al. Stress hormone and circulating biomarker profile of apical ballooning syndrome (takotsubo cardiomyopathy): insights into the clinical significance of B-type natriuretic peptide and troponin levels. Heart 2009; 95(17):1436–41.

51. Akashi YJ, Barbaro G, Sakurai T, et al. Cardiac autonomic imbalance in patients with reversible

ventricular dysfunction takotsubo cardiomyopathy. QJM 2007;100(6):335–43.

52. Ortak J, Khattab K, Barantke M, et al. Evolution of cardiac autonomic nervous activity indices in patients presenting with transient left ventricular apical ballooning. Pacing Clin Electrophysiol 2009;32(Suppl 1):S21–5.

53. Vaccaro A, Despas F, Delmas C, et al. Direct evidences for sympathetic hyperactivity and baroreflex impairment in tako tsubo cardiopathy. PLoS One 2014;9(3):e93278.

54. Sverrisdottir YB, Schultz T, Omerovic E, et al. Sympathetic nerve activity in stress-induced cardiomyopathy. Clin Auton Res 2012;22(6):259–64.

55. Akashi YJ, Nakazawa K, Sakakibara M, et al. 123I-MIBG myocardial scintigraphy in patients with "takotsubo" cardiomyopathy. J Nucl Med 2004; 45(7):1121–7.

56. Burgdorf C, von Hof K, Schunkert H, et al. Regional alterations in myocardial sympathetic innervation in patients with transient left-ventricular apical ballooning (Tako-Tsubo cardiomyopathy). J Nucl Cardiol 2008;15(1):65–72.

57. Cimarelli S, Sauer F, Morel O, et al. Transient left ventricular dysfunction syndrome: pathophysiological bases through nuclear medicine imaging. Int J Cardiol 2010;144(2):212–8.

58. Verberne HJ, van der Heijden DJ, van Eck-Smit BL, et al. Persisting myocardial sympathetic dysfunction in takotsubo cardiomyopathy. J Nucl Cardiol 2009;16(2):321–4.

59. Prasad A, Madhavan M, Chareonthaitawee P. Cardiac sympathetic activity in stress-induced (takotsubo) cardiomyopathy. Nat Rev Cardiol 2009;6(6):430–4.

60. Ueyama T, Kasamatsu K, Hano T, et al. Emotional stress induces transient left ventricular hypocontraction in the rat via activation of cardiac adrenoceptors: a possible animal model of 'tako-tsubo' cardiomyopathy. Circ J 2002; 66(7):712–3.

61. Izumi Y, Okatani H, Shiota M, et al. Effects of metoprolol on epinephrine-induced takotsubo-like left ventricular dysfunction in non-human primates. Hypertens Res 2009;32(5):339–46.

62. Paur H, Wright PT, Sikkel MB, et al. High levels of circulating epinephrine trigger apical cardiodepression in a beta2-adrenergic receptor/Gi-dependent manner: a new model of takotsubo cardiomyopathy. Circulation 2012;126(6):697–706.

63. Shao Y, Redfors B, Scharin Tang M, et al. Novel rat model reveals important roles of beta-adrenoreceptors in stress-induced cardiomyopathy. Int J Cardiol 2013;168(3):1943–50.

64. Redfors B, Ali A, Shao Y, et al. Different catecholamines induce different patterns of takotsubo-like cardiac dysfunction in an apparently afterload

dependent manner. Int J Cardiol 2014;174(2): 330–6.

65. Ibanez B, Navarro F, Farre J, et al. Tako-tsubo syndrome associated with a long course of the left anterior descending coronary artery along the apical diaphragmatic surface of the left ventricle. Rev Esp Cardiol 2004;57(3):209–16 [in Spanish].

66. Delgado GA, Truesdell AG, Kirchner RM, et al. An angiographic and intravascular ultrasound study of the left anterior descending coronary artery in takotsubo cardiomyopathy. Am J Cardiol 2011; 108(6):888–91.

67. Haghi D, Roehm S, Hamm K, et al. Takotsubo cardiomyopathy is not due to plaque rupture: an intravascular ultrasound study. Clin Cardiol 2010;33(5): 307–10.

68. Hoyt J, Lerman A, Lennon RJ, et al. Left anterior descending artery length and coronary atherosclerosis in apical ballooning syndrome (takotsubo/stress induced cardiomyopathy). Int J Cardiol 2010;145(1).112–5.

69. Angelini P. Transient left ventricular apical ballooning: a unifying pathophysiologic theory at the edge of Prinzmetal angina. Catheter Cardiovasc Interv 2008;71(3):342–52.

70. Angelini P, Monge J, Simpson L. Biventricular takotsubo cardiomyopathy: case report and general discussion. Tex Heart Inst J 2013;40(3):312–5.

71. Martinez-Selles M, Datino T, Pello AM, et al. Ergonovine provocative test in Caucasian patients with left ventricular apical ballooning syndrome. Int J Cardiol 2010;145(1):89–91.

72. Ghadri JR, Dougoud S, Maier W, et al. A PET/CT-follow-up imaging study to differentiate takotsubo cardiomyopathy from acute myocardial infarction. Int J Cardiovasc Imaging 2014;30(1): 207–9.

73. Meimoun P, Malaquin D, Sayah S, et al. The coronary flow reserve is transiently impaired in takotsubo cardiomyopathy: a prospective study using serial Doppler transthoracic echocardiography. J Am Soc Echocardiogr 2008;21(1):72–7.

74. Rigo F, Sicari R, Citro R, et al. Diffuse, marked, reversible impairment in coronary microcirculation in stress cardiomyopathy: a Doppler transthoracic echo study. Ann Med 2009;41(6):462–70.

75. Kume T, Akasaka T, Kawamoto T, et al. Assessment of coronary microcirculation in patients with takotsubo-like left ventricular dysfunction. Circ J 2005;69(8):934–9.

76. Bybee KA, Prasad A, Barsness GW, et al. Clinical characteristics and thrombolysis in myocardial infarction frame counts in women with transient left ventricular apical ballooning syndrome. Am J Cardiol 2004;94(3):343–6.

77. Elesber A, Lerman A, Bybee KA, et al. Myocardial perfusion in apical ballooning syndrome correlate

of myocardial injury. Am Heart J 2006;152(3):469. e9-13.

78. Uchida Y, Egami H, Uchida Y, et al. Possible participation of endothelial cell apoptosis of coronary microvessels in the genesis of takotsubo cardiomyopathy. Clin Cardiol 2010;33:371–7.

79. Vasilieva E, Vorobyeva I, Lebedeva A, et al. Brachial artery flow-mediated dilation in patients with tako-tsubo cardiomyopathy. Am J Med 2011; 124(12):1176–9.

80. Mann DL, Kent RL, Parsons B, et al. Adrenergic effects on the biology of the adult mammalian cardiocyte. Circulation 1992;85(2):790–804.

81. Nef HM, Mollmann H, Troidl C, et al. Abnormalities in intracellular Ca^{2+} regulation contribute to the pathomechanism of tako-tsubo cardiomyopathy. Eur Heart J 2009;30(17):2155–64.

82. Communal C, Colucci WS, Singh K. p38 mitogen-activated protein kinase pathway protects adult rat ventricular myocytes against beta -adrenergic receptor-stimulated apoptosis. Evidence for Gi-dependent activation. J Biol Chem 2000; 275(25):19395–400.

83. Nef HM, Mollmann H, Hilpert P, et al. Activated cell survival cascade protects cardiomyocytes from cell death in tako-tsubo cardiomyopathy. Eur J Heart Fail 2009;11(8):758–64.

84. Schultz T, Shao Y, Redfors B, et al. Stress-induced cardiomyopathy in Sweden: evidence for different ethnic predisposition and altered cardiocirculatory status. Cardiology 2012;122(3):180–6.

85. Lavi S, Nevo O, Thaler I, et al. Effect of aging on the cardiovascular regulatory systems in healthy women. Am J Physiol Regul Integr Comp Physiol 2007;292(2):R788–93.

86. Komesaroff PA, Esler MD, Sudhir K. Estrogen supplementation attenuates glucocorticoid and catecholamine responses to mental stress in perimenopausal women. J Clin Endocrinol Metab 1999;84(2):606–10.

87. Summers MR, Lennon RJ, Prasad A. Pre-morbid psychiatric and cardiovascular diseases in apical ballooning syndrome (tako-tsubo/stress-induced cardiomyopathy): potential pre-disposing factors? J Am Coll Cardiol 2010;55(7):700–1.

88. Delmas C, Lairez O, Mulin E, et al. Anxiodepressive disorders and chronic psychological stress are associated with tako-tsubo cardiomyopathy- new physiopathological hypothesis. Circ J 2013;77(1): 175–80.

89. Mausbach BT, Dimsdale JE, Ziegler MG, et al. Depressive symptoms predict norepinephrine response to a psychological stressor task in Alzheimer's caregivers. Psychosom Med 2005;67(4): 638–42.

90. Barton DA, Dawood T, Lambert EA, et al. Sympathetic activity in major depressive disorder: identifying those at increased cardiac risk? J Hypertens 2007;25(10):2117–24.

91. Alvarenga ME, Richards JC, Lambert G, et al. Psychophysiological mechanisms in panic disorder: a correlative analysis of noradrenaline spillover, neuronal noradrenaline reuptake, power spectral analysis of heart rate variability, and psychological variables. Psychosom Med 2006;68(1): 8–16.

92. Patel B, Assad D, Wiemann C, et al. Repeated use of albuterol inhaler as a potential cause of takotsubo cardiomyopathy. Am J Case Rep 2014;15: 221–5.

93. Amariles P, Cifuentes L. Drugs as possible triggers of takotsubo cardiomyopathy: a comprehensive literature search - update 2015. Curr Clin Pharmacol 2016;11:1–15.

94. Smeijers L, Szabo BM, van Dammen L, et al. Emotional, neurohormonal, and hemodynamic responses to mental stress in tako-tsubo cardiomyopathy. Am J Cardiol 2015;115(11):1580–6.

95. Norcliffe-Kaufmann L, Kaufmann H, Martinez J, et al. Autonomic findings in takotsubo cardiomyopathy. Am J Cardiol 2016;117(2):206–13.

96. Pereira VH, Marques P, Magalhaes R, et al. Central autonomic nervous system response to autonomic challenges is altered in patients with a previous episode of takotsubo cardiomyopathy. Eur Heart J Acute Cardiovasc Care 2015;5(2): 152–63.

97. Sader MA, Celermajer DS. Endothelial function, vascular reactivity and gender differences in the cardiovascular system. Cardiovasc Res 2002; 53(3):597–604.

98. Sung BH, Ching M, Izzo JL Jr, et al. Estrogen improves abnormal norepinephrine-induced vasoconstriction in postmenopausal women. J Hypertens 1999;17(4):523–8.

99. Sugimoto K, Inamasu J, Hirose Y, et al. The role of norepinephrine and estradiol in the pathogenesis of cardiac wall motion abnormality associated with subarachnoid hemorrhage. Stroke 2012; 43(7):1897–903.

100. Ueyama T, Ishikura F, Matsuda A, et al. Chronic estrogen supplementation following ovariectomy improves the emotional stress-induced cardiovascular responses by indirect action on the nervous system and by direct action on the heart. Circ J 2007;71(4):565–73.

101. Cao X, Zhou C, Chong J, et al. Estrogen resisted stress-induced cardiomyopathy through increasing the activity of beta(2)AR-Galphas signal pathway in female rats. Int J Cardiol 2015;187:377–86.

102. Barletta G, Del Pace S, Boddi M, et al. Abnormal coronary reserve and left ventricular wall motion during cold pressor test in patients with previous

left ventricular ballooning syndrome. Eur Heart J 2009;30(24):3007–14.

103. Martin EA, Prasad A, Rihal CS, et al. Endothelial function and vascular response to mental stress are impaired in patients with apical ballooning syndrome. J Am Coll Cardiol 2010;56(22):1840–6.

104. Patel SM, Lerman A, Lennon RJ, et al. Impaired coronary microvascular reactivity in women with apical ballooning syndrome (takotsubo/stress cardiomyopathy). Eur Heart J Acute Cardiovasc Care 2013;2(2):147–52.

105. Vriz O, Minisini R, Citro R, et al. Analysis of beta 1 and beta 2-adrenergic receptors polymorphism in patients with apical ballooning cardiomyopathy. Acta Cardiol 2011;66(6):787–90.

106. Sharkey SW, Maron BJ, Nelson P, et al. Adrenergic receptor polymorphisms in patients with stress

(tako-tsubo) cardiomyopathy. J Cardiol 2009; 53(1):53–7.

107. Spinelli L, Trimarco V, Di Marino S, et al. L41Q polymorphism of the G protein coupled receptor kinase 5 is associated with left ventricular apical ballooning syndrome. Eur J Heart Fail 2010;12(1): 13–6.

108. Novo G, Giambanco S, Guglielmo M, et al. G-protein-coupled receptor kinase 5 polymorphism and takotsubo cardiomyopathy. J Cardiovasc Med 2014;16(9):639–43.

109. Figtree GA, Bagnall RD, Abdulla I, et al. No association of G-protein-coupled receptor kinase 5 or beta-adrenergic receptor polymorphisms with takotsubo cardiomyopathy in a large Australian cohort. Eur J Heart Fail 2013;15(7): 730–3.

Genetics of Takotsubo Syndrome

Giuseppe Limongelli, MD, PhD, FESC[a,*], Daniele Masarone, MD[a], Valeria Maddaloni, MD[b], Marta Rubino, MD[a], Fiorella Fratta, MD[a], Annapaola Cirillo, MD[a], Spinelli Barrile Ludovica, MD[a], Roberta Pacileo, MD[a], Adelaide Fusco, MD[a], Guido Ronald Coppola, MD[a], Francesca Pisacane, MD[a], Eduardo Bossone, MD, PhD, FCCP, FESC, FACC[c,d], Paolo Calabrò, MD, PhD, FESC[a], Raffaele Calabrò, MD[a], Maria Giovanna Russo, MD[a], Giuseppe Pacileo, MD[a]

KEYWORDS

- Takotsubo syndrome • Catecholamine-induced myocardial toxicity • Adrenoceptor polymorphisms

KEY POINTS

- Takotsubo syndrome (TTS) is an enigmatic disease with a multifactorial and still unresolved pathogenesis.
- A genetic predisposition has been suggested based on the few familial TTS cases described.
- Conflicting results have been published regarding the role of functional polymorphisms in relevant candidate genes, such as α_1-, β_1-, and β_2-adrenergic receptors; G protein–coupled receptor kinase 5 (GRK5); and estrogen receptors.
- Further research is required to help clarify the role of genetic susceptibility in TTS.

INTRODUCTION

During the past 2 decades, a novel cardiac syndrome with transient left ventricular systolic dysfunction has been reported.[1,2] Often referred to as TTS, owing to the shape and appearance of the left ventricle at end systole resembling a Japanese octopus fishing pot during the acute phase, this disorder is also termed, stress cardiomyopathy, apical ballooning, and broken heart syndrome.[3] TTS syndrome is classified as both a primary and an acquired cardiomyopathy by the American Heart Association[3] and as an unclassified cardiomyopathy by the European Society of Cardiology.[4,5] Whether this disorder represents a true cardiomyopathy remains to be determined.

In the meantime, according to recent article from the Heart Failure Association of the European Society of Cardiology,[6] this entity should be clinically labeled an "acute, reversible, heart failure syndrome." The cause of TTS remains subject of investigation—observational data in patients with subarachnoid hemorrhage,[7] reports of its occurrence in patients with pheochromocytoma, and its reproduction by infusion of epinephrine in primates[8] strongly support the hypothesis that it is caused by excessive adrenergic/catecholamine stimulation.[9] Moreover, recent evidence has suggested a genetic role in TTS.[10] This review discusses the role of genetics, in particular adrenoceptor polymorphisms, in the pathobiology of TTS.

DEFINITION OF TAKOTSUBO SYNDROME

Diagnostic criteria for TTS have been proposed from several centers, using various diagnostic

[a] Cardiologia SUN, Monaldi Hospital, AORN dei Colli, Second University of Naples, Via L Bianchi, Naples 80100, Italy; [b] Genomic and Cellular Lab, Monaldi Hospital, AORN dei Colli, Second University of Naples, Via L Bianchi, Naples 80100, Italy; [c] Heart Department, University Hospital "San Giovanni di Dio e Ruggi d'Aragona", Salerno, Italy; [d] Cardiology Division, Heart Department, "Cava de' Tirreni and Amalfi Coast" Hospital, University of Salerno, via De Marinis, Cava de" Tirreni (SA) 84013, Italy
* Corresponding author.
E-mail address: limongelligiuseppe@libero.it

Heart Failure Clin 12 (2016) 499–506
http://dx.doi.org/10.1016/j.hfc.2016.06.007
1551-7136/16/© 2016 Elsevier Inc. All rights reserved.

definitions.[6,11,12] A detailed description of the diverse definitions is behind the scope of this review; however, **Box 1** summarizes the diagnostic criteria more frequently used in clinical practice.

PATHOPHYSIOLOGY OF TAKOTSUBO SYNDROME

The pathophysiology of TTS is complex and reflects the integrated and systemic physiologic responses to stress and the cardiovascular responses to sudden surges of catecholamines.[13]

Several hypotheses have been proposed to explain the unique cardiac appearance in TTS and the cardiac response to severe stress.[14] Many of these hypotheses are still being investigated, because there is no current proved pathophysiologic mechanism to explain TTS (**Box 2**). The prevailing mechanistic hypothesis, however, invokes catecholamine surge-induced cardiac toxicity.

Support for a possible pathogenic role for catecholamines comes from studies in which plasma catecholamines were measured at presentation. Wittstein and colleagues[15] found that the serum

---

Box 1
Diagnostic criteria for Takotsubo syndrome

Mayo Clinic modified criteria (Prasad and colleagues,[11] 2008)

Transient hypokinesis, dyskinesis, or akinesis of the left ventricular midsegments, with or without apical involvement; the regional wall motion abnormalities extend beyond a single epicardial vascular distribution, and a stressful trigger is often, but not always, present

New ECG abnormalities (either ST-segment elevation and/or T-wave inversion) or modest elevation in cardiac troponin level

Absence of obstructive coronary disease or angiographic evidence of acute plaque rupture

Absence of pheochromocytoma or myocarditis

Italian Network criteria (Parodi and colleagues,[12] 2014)

Typical transient left ventricular wall motion abnormalities extending beyond a single epicardial vascular distribution with complete functional normalization within 6 weeks

Absence of potentially culprit coronary stenosis or angiographic evidence of acute plaque rupture, dissection, thrombosis, or spasm

New and dynamic ST-segment abnormalities or T-wave inversion as well as new onset of transient or permanent left bundle branch block

Mild increase in myocardial injury markers (creatine kinase-MB value <50 U/L)

Clinical and/or instrumental exclusion of myocarditis

Postmenopausal woman (optional)

Antecedent stressful event (optional)

Heart Failure Association criteria (Lyon and colleagues,[6] 2016)

Transient regional wall motion abnormalities of left ventricle or right ventricle, which are frequently, but not always, preceded by a stressful trigger (emotional or physical)

The regional wall motion abnormalities usually extend beyond a single epicardial vascular distribution and often result in circumferential dysfunction of the ventricular segments involved.

The absence of culprit atherosclerotic coronary artery disease, including acute plaque rupture, thrombus formation, and coronary dissection or other pathologic conditions to explain the pattern of temporary left ventricle dysfunction observed (eg, hypertrophic cardiomyopathy and viral myocarditis)

New and reversible ECG abnormalities (ST-segment elevation, ST depression, left bundle branch block, T-wave inversion, and/or QTc prolongation) during the acute phase (3 months)

Significantly elevated serum natriuretic peptide (brain natriuretic peptide or N-terminal prohormone of brain natriuretic peptide) during the acute phase

Positive but small elevation in cardiac troponin measured with a conventional assay (ie, disparity between the troponin level and the amount of dysfunctional myocardium present)

Recovery of ventricular systolic function on cardiac imaging at follow-up (3–6 months)

Box 2
Summary of proposed pathophysiologic hypothesis and of predisposing factors for Takotsubo syndrome

Pathophysiologic hypothesis

Catecholamine-mediated myocardial stunning

Multivessel epicardial coronary artery spasm

Coronary microvascular dysfunction

Left ventricular outflow tract obstruction and abnormal left ventricular arterial coupling

Acute atherosclerotic plaque rupture in the left anterior descending coronary artery

Predisposing factors

Postmenopausal hormonal status

Thrombophilic status

Genetic polymorphism

---

catecholamine concentration was 2 to 3 times greater in patients with TTS than that in patients with acute coronary syndrome. It has been reported that exogenously administered catecholamines,[16] pheochromocytoma,[17] and acute brain injury[18] cause similar reversible myocardial dysfunction.

In addition, myocardial biopsies of patients with TTS demonstrate typical features of catecholamine toxicity (accumulation of glycogen in cytoplasm of myocytes, disorganization of contractile and cytoskeletal proteins, and an increased extracellular matrix), which are nearly complete reversible at 2 weeks,[19] and the peculiar distribution of the condition may be explained by the greater adrenergic beta-receptor subtype density at the apex of the heart in comparison with the basal myocardium.[8,20,21]

Multiple mechanisms have been postulated to explain the cardiotoxicity of catecholamines.[22] The overstimulation of catecholamine receptors enhances cardiac contractility and heart rate, with a secondary increase in myocardial oxygen demand that may outweigh oxygen delivery, creating areas of functional hypoxia that can be exacerbated by vasoconstriction in the coronary macrocirculation and microcirculation and that reduce the supply of high-energy phosphates.[23] This picture can be further aggravated by metabolic changes, such as the stimulation of lipolysis with deposition of neutral lipid droplets in cardiomyocytes, resulting in an uncoupling of oxidative phosphorylation.[24] Changes in membrane permeability leading to various electrolytic imbalances disturb multiple cellular homeostatic processes, fostering additional myocardial toxicity.[25]

ROLE OF GENETICS IN TAKOTSUBO SYNDROME

The trigger of clinical events in TTS is commonly a "stressful event", and this is consistent with a strong "environmental component" in this patients. It is conceivable, however, that some people have a genetic predisposition to TTS. Genetic underpinnings for TTS are supported by several lines of reasoning.

First, 3 case reports document familial TTS in a mother-daughter pair[26] and 2 sister pairs.[27,28] Second, most postmenopausal women experience acute stressful events, yet only a small subset develops TTS. Third, 20% of patients report no preceding stressor,[29] and some women have TTS episodes prior to menopause, implicating an intrinsic pathogenic mechanism not solely dependent on hormonal environment. Fourth, TTS recurs in 11% of patients,[30] strongly suggesting genetically mediated vulnerability.

Over the past decade, several studies analyzing polymorphisms potentially involved in the pathogenesis of TTS have been published (**Table 1**), the most important of which concern those affecting adrenergic receptors located on cell membranes, which exist as several subtypes (α_1, α_2, β_1, β_2, and β_3).[31]

The intracellular signaling after catecholamine binding to the receptor is mediated by adrenergic receptors β_1 and β_2, which couple to the G alpha subunit of the Gs protein complex. At the same time, catecholamines induce phosphorylation of G protein–coupled receptor kinase to negatively regulate the signal.[32] Common genetic polymorphisms in beta-receptor subtypes include Arg389 and Ser49 in the adrenergic receptor subtype β_1 (ADRB1). The first has been proposed to lead to functional alteration of the Gs protein-coupling domain, and the presence of the arginine instead of glycine in the second is predicted to cause a gain of function of the encoded protein. Polymorphisms in the gene encoding the adrenergic receptor α_{2C} (ADRA2C) (a receptor that regulates norepinephrine release from sympathetic cardiac nerves gene) may cause adrenergic deregulation. In particular, a deletion of 4 amino acids (protein positions from 322 to 325) causes an impairment of receptor coupling, leading to an alteration of the signaling to inhibition of adenylyl cyclase, stimulation of inositol phosphate accumulation, and activation of mitogen-activated protein kinase. This polymorphism has been found more frequently in African American than in white patients, and its functional consequence can cause an increased response to antagonists compared with wild-type carriers, with a possible modification in drug response and disease development of

Table 1
Summary of polymorphisms found in patients affected by Takotsubo cardiomyopathy

Protein Name	Gene Symbol	SNP Identification	Protein Variation	Genetic Polymorphism	Effect	Results: Patient
β_1-Adrenergic receptor	ADRB1	rs1801253 rs1801252 rs1801253	Gly389ArgSer-49GlyArg31Gln	—	Enhanced cardiac catecholamine sensitivity	Gly389ArgHomozygous for 389-Arg:44-y-old woman with familial ABS3049% homozygous for Arg-389, 49% heterozygous, 2% homozygous for Gly-38930Homozygous for 389-Arg 42%, homozygous for 389-Gly 12%, heterozygous 47% 31Arg31GlnNonsignificant difference between patients and controls32Ser49GlyHomozygous for 49-Ser:44-y-old woman with familial ABS3088% homozygous for Ser-49, 12% heterozygous[33]
β_2-Adrenergic receptor	ADRB2	rs1042713 rs1042714 rs1800888	Arg16GlyGln27GluThr164Ile	—	Possible increased vulnerability of the heart to adrenergic stress	Arg16GlyWild type:44-y-old woman with familial ABS31 and 34Homozygous for Arg-16 13%, homozygous for Gly-16 28%, heterozygous 59% Gln27GluHomozygous for Gln-27 10%, homozygous for Glu-27 38%, heterozygous 52% 35Thr164IleNonsignificant difference between patients and controls[31]

α$_{2C}$-Adrenergic receptor	ADRA2C	rs2234888	del322–325	—	Impaired regulation of norepinephrine release	Wild type (no deletion):44-y-old woman with familial ABS3293% wild type; 7% heterozygous34Nonsignificant difference between patients and controls[30]
Fragile X mental retardation	FMR1	—	Reduction of gene expression	Insertion of CGG trinucleotide	Fragile X syndrome	Female patient carrying the mutation[33]
Gs-protein α subunit	GNAS	rs11554276	—	g.56503898G>A	—	Nonsignificant difference between patients and controls[32]
G protein–coupled receptor kinase 5	GRK5	rs17098707 rs34679178	Gln41LeuThr129Met	—	—	Gln41LeuDifferent distribution of Gln41Leu between takotsubo patients and controls; leucine34 associated with lower heart rate in the female portion of the population32Thr129MetNonsignificant difference between patients and controls[32]
CD36	CD36	rs75326924	P90S	c.268C>TIns1159A	CD36 deficiency	One patient with TTC described with both heterozygous variations[32]

Abbreviation: SNP, single nucleotide polymorphism.

From Limongelli G, D'Alessandro R, Masarone D, et al. Takotsubo cardiomyopathy: do the genetics matter? Heart Fail Clin 2013;9(2):212–3; with permission.

deletion carriers.[33] Animal model studies suggest the involvement of adrenergic receptor β_2 in stress-induced cardiomyopathy, because an increased concentration of such receptors has been found in the apical region of dog hearts. In mice models, the overexpression of receptors belonging to the subtype β_2 in the apical region of the heart has been found associated with increased levels of epinephrine. Together, these data suggest that when stress events occur, the increase in circulating epinephrine can have a major effect on the apical region of the heart because of a difference in sensitivity of β_2 receptors.[14]

In a cohort of 61 white patients (58 women, 95%; mean age 69 + 11 years) with TTS, Sharkey and colleagues[34] found no difference in the frequency of adrenoceptor ADRA2C and adrenoceptor ADRB1 polymorphisms compared with controls, whereas Vriz and colleagues[35] found a different distribution of variation of β_1 (Arg389Gly; homozygous Arg/Arg more frequent in TTS) and β2 (Gln27Glu; homozygous Gln/Gln more frequent in healthy controls) adrenergic receptors among patients and controls but no significant difference for β_2-adrenergic receptor (Arg16Gly) variation.

Spinelli and colleagues[36] investigated the presence of genetic polymorphisms in ADRB1, ADRB2, Gs-protein α subunit (GNAS), GRK5 genes in 22 patients, 21 of whom had a stressful event as an ascertained cause of TTS. The genetic analysis showed a similar distribution between cases and controls for most of the polymorphisms but a significant difference for the polymorphism rs17098707 in the GRK5 gene, with a higher prevalence among TTS subjects. The association between the polymorphism and the cardiac phenotype could be explained by the negative inotropic effect of the GRK5 L41 variant under conditions of acute catecholamine stimulation.

A whole-exome sequencing for genes related to catecholamines and adrenergic signaling was recently carried out on 28 TTS patients, including a mother-daughter pair and 5 recurrent cases.[37] Investigators identified malignant variants in 55 candidate genes and no homozygous or compound heterozygous mutations and, therefore, excluded a recessive transmissibility in these patients; among these, 7 genes were common variants in more than 1 patient in the population analyzed. Approximately 93% of the patients had at least a malignant variant, and the finding of the same variants in the control population could be readily accepted by having the basic information of how the environmental influence is decisive in the development of this phenotype.

Other investigators focused their attention on a particular aspect of the Takotsubo phenotype. In 2013, Citro and colleagues[38] focused on impaired endothelium-dependent vasodilation, excessive vasoconstriction, and increased sympathetic activation after acute mental stress observed in TTS patients. They analyzed a population of 29 patients and more than 1000 healthy controls for the presence of mutations in the protein Bcl2-associated BCL2 associated athanogene 3 (BAG3). This protein is expressed in only a few cell types, including cardiomyocytes: among its functions, it mediates the cellular response to stress.

Given the extremely low power for studies of this size in detecting an effect of a common polymorphism, further studies with high-quality phenotyping and sharing high-number/high-quality data in a TTS network are necessary to estimate the potential role of the genetics as a predisposing factor in TTS.

SUMMARY

TTS is an enigmatic disease with a multifactorial and still unresolved pathogenesis. Conflicting results have been published regarding the presence or absence of functional polymorphisms in relevant candidate genes, such as α_1-, β_1-, and β_2-adrenergic receptors; GRK5; and estrogen receptors. Resolving these conflicts through high-quality phenotyping, identification of candidate genes, and sharing of high-number/high-quality data in a TTS network will shed new light on understanding the pathogenesis of this peculiar syndrome.

REFERENCES

1. Sato H, Taiteishi H, Uchida T. Takotsubo-type cardiomyopathy due to multivessel spasm. In: Kodama K, Haze K, Hon M, editors. Clinical aspect of myocardial injury: from ischemia to heart failure. Tokyo (Japan): Kagakuhyouronsha; 1990. p. 56.

2. Dote K, Sato H, Tateishi H, et al. Myocardial stunning due to simultaneous multivessel coronary spasms: a review of 5 cases. J Cardiol 1991;21: 203–10.

3. Bybee KA, Kara T, Prasad A, et al. Systematic review: transient left ventricular apical ballooning: a syndrome that mimics ST-segment elevation myocardial infarction. Ann Intern Med 2004;141: 858–63.

4. Maron BJ, Towbin JA, Thiene G, et al. Contemporary definitions and classification of the cardiomyopathies: an American Heart Association Scientific Statement from the Council on Clinical Cardiology, Heart Failure and Transplantation Committee; Quality of Care and Outcomes Research and Functional Genomics and Translational Biology Interdisciplinary

Working Groups; and Council on Epidemiology and Prevention. Circulation 2006;113:1807–16.

5. Elliott P, Andersson B, Arbustini E, et al. Classification of the cardiomyopathies: a position statement from the European Society Of Cardiology Working Group on Myocardial and Pericardial Diseases. Eur Heart J 2008;29:270–88.

6. Lyon AR, Bossone E, Schneider B, et al. Current state of knowledge on Takotsubo syndrome: a position Statement from the Taskforce on Takotsubo Syndrome of the Heart Failure Association of the European Society of Cardiology. Eur J Heart Fail 2016;18:8–27.

7. Ako J, Sudhir K, Farouque HM, et al. Transient left ventricular dysfunction under severe stress: brain-heart relationship revisited. Am J Med 2006;119:10–7.

8. Paur H, Wright PT, Sikkel MB, et al. High levels of circulating epinephrine trigger apical cardiodepression in a β2-adrenergic receptor/Gi-dependent manner: a new model of Takotsubo cardiomyopathy. Circulation 2012;126:697–705.

9. Kassim TA, Clarke DD, Mai VQ, et al. Catecholamine-induced cardiomyopathy. Endocr Pract 2008;14:1137–43.

10. Limongelli G, D'Alessandro R, Masarone D, et al. Takotsubo cardiomyopathy: do the genetics matter? Heart Fail Clin 2013;9:207–16.

11. Prasad A, Lerman A, Rihal CS. Apical ballooning syndrome (Tako-Tsubo or stress cardiomyopathy): a mimic of acute myocardial infarction. Am Heart J 2008;155:408–17.

12. Parodi G, Citro R, Bellandi B, et al. Tako-tsubo Italian Network (TIN). Revised clinical diagnostic criteria for Tako-tsubo syndrome: the Tako-tsubo Italian Network proposal. Int J Cardiol 2014;172:282–7.

13. Akashi YJ, Nef HM, Lyon AR. Epidemiology and pathophysiology of Takotsubo syndrome. Nat Rev Cardiol 2015;12:387–9.

14. Lyon AR, Rees PS, Prasad S, et al. Stress (Takotsubo) cardiomyopathy–a novel pathophysiological hypothesis to explain catecholamine-induced acute myocardial stunning. Nat Clin Pract Cardiovasc Med 2008;5:22–8.

15. Wittstein IS, Thiemann DR, Lima JA, et al. Neurohumoral features of myocardial stunning due to sudden emotional stress. N Engl J Med 2005;352:539–48.

16. Abraham J, Mudd JO, Kapur NK, et al. Stress cardiomyopathy after intravenous administration of catecholamines and beta-receptor agonists. J Am Coll Cardiol 2009;53:1320–5.

17. Bravo EL, Tagle R. Pheochromocytoma: state-of-the-art and future prospects. Endocr Rev 2003;24:539–53.

18. Grunsfeld A, Fletcher JJ, Nathan BR. Cardiopulmonary complications of brain injury. Curr Neurol Neurosci Rep 2005;5:488–93.

19. Ueda H, Hosokawa Y, Tsujii U, et al. An autopsy case of left ventricular apical ballooning probably caused by pheochromocytoma with persistent ST-segment elevation. Int J Cardiol 2011;149:50–2.

20. Meimoun P, Passos P, Benali T, et al. Assessment of left ventricular twist mechanics in Tako-tsubo cardiomyopathy by two-dimensional speckle-tracking echocardiography. Eur J Echocardiogr 2011;12:931–9.

21. Pacileo G, Baldini L, Limongelli G, et al. Prolonged left ventricular twist in cardiomyopathies: a potential link between systolic and diastolic dysfunction. Eur J Echocardiogr 2011;12:841–9.

22. Liaudet L, Calderari B, Pacher P. Pathophysiological mechanisms of catecholamine and cocaine-mediated cardiotoxicity. Heart Fail Rev 2014;1:815–24.

23. Zhang X, Szeto C, Gao E, et al. Cardiotoxic and cardioprotective features of chronic b-adrenergic signaling. Circ Res 2008;112:498–509.

24. Behonick GS, Novak MJ, Nealley EW, et al. Toxicology update: the cardiotoxicity of the oxidative stress metabolites of catecholamines (aminochromes). J Appl Toxicol 2001;21:15–S22.

25. Borkowski BJ, Cheema Y, Shahbaz AU, et al. Cation dyshomeostasis and cardiomyocyte necrosis: the Fleckenstein hypothesis revisited. Eur Heart J 2001;32:1846–53.

26. Kumar G, Holmes D Jr, Prasad A. 'Familial' apical ballooning syndrome (Takotsubocardiomyopathy). Int J Cardiol 2009;44:444–5.

27. Pison L, De Vusser P, Mullens W. Apical ballooning in relatives. Heart 2004;90:e67.

28. Ikutomi M, Yamasaki M, Matsusita M, et al. Takotsubo cardiomyopathy in siblings. Heart Vessels 2014;29:119–22.

29. Pilgrim TM, Wyss TR. Takotsubo cardiomyopathy or transient left ventricular apical ballooning syndrome: a systematic review. Int J Cardiol 2008;124:283–92.

30. Elesber AA, Prasad A, Lennon RJ, et al. Four-year recurrence rate and prognosis of the apical ballooning syndrome. J Am Coll Cardiol 2007;50:448–52.

31. Workman AJ. Cardiac adrenergic control and atrial fibrillation. Naunyn Schmiedebergs Arch Pharmacol 2010;381:235–49.

32. Dorn GW 2nd. Adrenergic signaling polymorphisms and their impact on cardiovascular disease. Physiol Rev 2010;90:1013–62.

33. Small KM, Forbes SL, Rahman FF, et al. A four amino acid deletion polymorphism in the third intracellular loop of the human alpha 2C-adrenergic receptor confers impaired coupling to multiple effectors. J Biol Chem 2000;275:23059–64.

34. Sharkey SW, Maron BJ, Nelson P, et al. Adrenergic receptor polymorphisms in patients with stress (takotsubo) cardiomyopathy. J Cardiol 2009;53:53–7.

35. Vriz O, Minisini R, Citro R, et al. Analysis of beta1 and beta2-adrenergic receptors polymorphism in patients with apical ballooning cardiomyopathy. Acta Cardiol 2011;66:787–90.

36. Spinelli L, Trimarco V, Di Marino S, et al. L41Q polymorphism of the G protein coupled receptor kinase 5 is associated with left ventricular apical ballooning syndrome. Eur J Heart Fail 2010;12:13–6.

37. Goodloe AH, Evans JM, Middha S, et al. Characterizing genetic variation of adrenergic signalling pathways in Takotsubo (stress) cardiomyopathy exomes. Eur J Heart Fail 2014;16:942–9.

38. Citro R, D'Avenia M, De Marco M, et al. Polymorphisms of the antiapoptotic protein bag3 may play a role in the pathogenesis of tako-tsubo cardiomyopathy. Int J Cardiol 2013;168:1663–5.

A Clinical Perspective of the Takotsubo Syndrome

Scott W. Sharkey, MD

KEYWORDS

- Takotsubo syndrome • Stress cardiomyopathy • Apical ballooning

KEY POINTS

- Takotsubo syndrome (TTS) is a unique form of acute myocardial injury with visually distinctive left ventricular (LV) contraction profile, predilection for women greater than 50 years of age, association with a triggering stressful event, and is typically completely reversible.
- At presentation, TTS closely resembles acute coronary syndrome with symptoms of chest pain or dyspnea, ischemic ECG changes, and troponin elevation. Abnormal LV contraction is in a noncoronary distribution and is independent of acute epicardial coronary obstruction.
- Recognition of TTS is increasing. The condition may present as a primary event with predominantly cardiac symptoms or as a secondary event in a health care–related setting during evaluation or treatment of a major illness.
- Complications include acute decompensated heart failure, acute mitral valve regurgitation, ventricular arrhythmias including cardiac arrest, LV outflow tract obstruction, and ventricular mural thrombi with embolization potential.
- Hospital mortality is 3% to 5%, posthospital survival is less than the general population, and recurrence rate is 5% to 10%. Complete recovery of LV systolic function is a TTS hallmark. β-Blockers do not prevent TTS occurrence and do not necessarily improve long-term outcome.

INTRODUCTION

In the course of 25 years, the TTS has emerged as an important form of acute myocardial injury characterized by distinctive regional LV contraction failure, often with marked reduction of LV ejection fraction, and is typically completely reversible. The original description in 1990 included 5 patients and was published in Japanese[1]; consequently, TTS remained largely unknown outside of Japan until the late 1990s when publications emerged in the English literature.[2] Thereafter, TTS became internationally recognized with greater than 1000 reports by 2011.[3–10]

At presentation TTS is often indistinguishable from acute coronary syndrome, yet its occurrence is independent of epicardial coronary artery obstruction.[11–14] Other features include a predilection for older women and association with antecedent stressful event. With greater recognition, the prevalence has increased (approximately 5%–10% of women with suspected acute coronary syndrome) and TTS now represents an important cause of acute heart failure (**Fig. 1**).[15,16] In the early experience, typical patients were older women, with a triggering emotional event, ST-segment elevation, and apical ballooning LV contraction pattern. Now, TTS is more clinically varied, recognized in men and younger individuals, without ST-segment elevation, as a spontaneous event without a trigger and with anatomically diverse LV contraction patterns beyond the classic apical ballooning type.[2–14,17] TTS is also associated with a far greater spectrum of emotional or

Disclosures/Conflict of Interest: None.
Cardiovascular Research Division, Minneapolis Heart Institute Foundation, 920 East 28th Street, Suite 620, Minneapolis, MN 55407, USA
E-mail address: scott.sharkey@allina.com

Heart Failure Clin 12 (2016) 507–520
http://dx.doi.org/10.1016/j.hfc.2016.06.003

heartfailure.theclinics.com

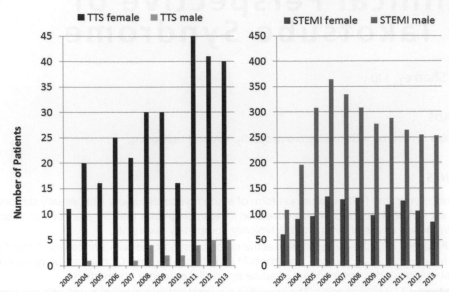

Fig. 1. Number of patients with TTS compared with STEMI. Tabulated by year from 2003 to 2013 at Minneapolis Heart Institute. TTS patients: black Indicates women (n = 295), green are men (n = 24); STEMI patients: red indicates women (n = 1173), blue are men (n = 2954). (*Adapted from* Sharkey SW. Epidemiology and clinical profile of Takotsubo cardiomyopathy. Circ J 2014;78:2120; with permission.)

physical triggers, including presentation during medical diagnostic procedures, outpatient treatment, or hospitalization for acute illness.[13,14] Although TTS has been considered a benign condition, it now carries a small but important risk for adverse outcomes. Hemodynamic instability requiring intervention with vasopressor drugs or intra-aortic balloon pump (IABP) is necessary in 15%, and in-hospital mortality is 3% to 5%, largely due to refractory cardiogenic shock or irreversible major comorbid conditions.[18,19] Despite complete and often rapid cardiac recovery, posthospital survival may be less than in the general population of similar age, largely because of concomitant illnesses.[11,18] TTS recurrence rate is 5% to 10%, but β-blocking drugs are not absolutely preventive for a TTS event and do not necessarily promote a more favorable outcome.

CLINICAL CONSIDERATIONS
Diagnostic Criteria

Specific diagnostic criteria have been proposed and refined over time,[20,21] including those recently published by the European Society of Cardiology (**Box 1**).[14] A persuasive argument has been made for using the term, *takotsubo syndrome*, rather than *takotsubo cardiomyopathy*, to describe this condition.[14] No single feature distinguishes TTS from other cardiac conditions with a similar acute presentation, such as coronary syndrome or myocarditis. Hallmark characteristics include

visually distinctive LV contraction abnormalities in a noncoronary distribution, absence of acute coronary artery obstruction or plaque rupture, and reversibility. For the clinician, the most challenging task is distinguishing TTS from acute

---

Box 1
Diagnostic features of takotsubo syndrome

- Acute onset as a primary event, or secondary event in the setting of major illness, commonly with antecedent stressful trigger

- Abnormal LV contraction anatomically inconsistent with a major coronary artery distribution. Discrete variants include apical ballooning (abnormal apical and midventricular segments), midventricular ballooning (abnormal midventricular segments), and inverted ballooning (abnormal basal ventricular segments)

- Absence of plaque rupture or severe stenosis in a coronary artery corresponding to region of abnormal LV contraction, bystander obstructive coronary artery disease does not exclude the diagnosis

- Ischemic ECG abnormality and troponin elevation, cases with normal ECG and troponin have been reported.

- Reversibility with demonstration of normal LV wall motion and ejection fraction at follow-up, typically within 1 to 3 months

coronary syndrome and, to a lesser extent, acute myocarditis.

Presentation

In general, TTS has a sudden onset with symptoms (chest discomfort and dyspnea) or signs of myocardial injury (heart failure, arrhythmia, ECG abnormality, and troponin elevation), commonly with an antecedent trigger. Patients usually present with 1 of 2 distinct clinical scenarios, that is, as a principal event with onset of cardiac symptoms at home or in the community or, alternatively,

as a secondary event in a health care–related setting during evaluation or treatment of an illness[13,14,16,22] (**Table 1**). This distinction is relevant, with major differences in patient characteristics and implications for outcome.

Patients with TTS as a principal event generally present to an emergency department with chest pain or dyspnea, symptoms that are often indistinguishable from acute coronary syndrome.[23,24] Consequently, these patients are usually admitted to a specialized cardiac unit and are usually initially treated with aspirin and anticoagulants.

Table 1
Clinical features of takotsubo syndrome

Attribute	Comment
Acute onset	Frequent
Presentation with acute chest pain or dyspnea	TTS as primary event in emergency department setting
Presentation in hospital with abnormal ECG, troponin elevation, hypotension, arrhythmia, heart failure	TTS as secondary event in context of major illness
Female gender[a]	90%
Age	Average age 65 y
Antecedant physical stressor[a]	30%–40%
Antecedant emotional stressor[a]	30%–40%
Antecedant stressor absent	10%–20%
ST-segment elevation on initial ECG	40%–50%, often indistinguishable from anterior STEMI
Evolution to T-wave inversion with QTc lengthening	Very frequent
Troponin release	90%, peak usually <1 ng/mL
LV systolic dysfunction	Ejection fraction typically 30%–40%, often <25%
Apical ballooning[a]	75%–80%
Midventricular ballooning	10%–20%
Inverted ballooning	<5%
CMR imaging late gadolinium enhancement	Rare
Acute pulmonary edema or cardiogenic shock	10%–15%
Hypotension requiring IABP	15%
RV involvement	20%–30%
LV outflow tract obstruction	10%–20%
Mitral regurgitation ≥ moderate	15%–20%
LV or RV thrombus	5%
Reversible LV dysfunction (stunning)[a]	Generally within 1–2 wk, rapid (48 h) or delayed (3 mo)
Hospital death	3%–5%
Recurrence	5%–10%
Ventricular fibrillation, pulseless electrical activity, asystole	<5%
Torsades de pointes ventricular tachycardia	Rare

[a] Considered a hallmark of the condition.

In contrast, secondary TTS often presents insidiously within a variety of health care settings, such as during surgical procedures (eg, orthopedic, abdominal, neurologic, cosmetic, and cardiac), with acute medical conditions (eg, sepsis, stroke, malignancy, acute respiratory failure, and trauma), or during outpatient procedures (eg, endoscopy, tissue biopsy, chemotherapy, and stress testing). In these situations, TTS may manifest itself atypically with arrhythmia, hypotension, acute pulmonary edema, abnormal ECG, or troponin elevation.[25,26] With an aging population and greater illness severity in hospitalized patients, secondary TTS will no doubt expand. A recent analysis of US Medicare data revealed a 3-fold increase in the discharge diagnosis of TTS, with much of the increase within the subgroup of patients with TTS as a secondary diagnosis.[16]

Diversity of Triggering Events

An intriguing TTS feature is its frequent association with an antecedent stressful event. In early reports, these events were largely related to emotional trauma.[3–8] As experience has expanded, a greater association with physical stressors has emerged.[13,14,18,19,23] Examples include intravenous chemotherapy for lung cancer, gastric ulcer with hemorrhage, intracranial bleeding, septic shock from intestinal perforation, and exacerbation of chronic obstructive pulmonary disease. TTS may also occur without an identifiable trigger in a substantial minority of patients, which has called into question the appropriateness of the moniker "stress cardiomyopathy" for the overall condition.[10] In the Minneapolis Heart Institute experience of approximately 400 TTS patients, 10% provided no history of a triggering event, physical stressors were present in 50%, and emotional events were present in 40%. Over time, an emergence of physical events and decline in emotional events have been observed as identified TTS triggers. In comparison, a report from the International Takotsubo Registry[19] noted triggering events as physical in 36%, emotional in 28%, both in 8%, and none in 29%. The increased association with a physical trigger likely reflects greater awareness of secondary TTS complicating acute illness.

The diversity of triggering events associated with TTS is remarkable and ranges from the catastrophic to the ordinary.[13,14,19,27] Several reports have linked TTS with conditions known to produce high circulating catecholamine levels, including pheochromocytoma and paraganglioma.[28,29] Catecholamine administration (epinephrine or dobutamine) in both therapeutic and excessive doses has also been associated with TTS onset.[30] These observations further support the hypothesis that elevated catecholamine levels may be involved in TTS pathophysiology.[7]

ECG Spectrum

No ECG characteristic reliably distinguishes TTS from acute coronary syndrome. The initial 12-lead ECG is abnormal in most TTS patients, usually with ischemic ST-segment and T-wave changes.[13,14] In 40% to 50% of cases, ST-segment elevation is present in the precordial leads in a pattern indistinguishable from that of acute anterior myocardial infarction due to left anterior descending (LAD) coronary artery occlusion (**Fig. 2**). Although some investigators have proposed ECG criteria for differentiating the ST-segment elevation observed in TTS from that of acute LAD occlusion, the diagnostic accuracy is insufficient for clinical use.[31,32] Other ECG patterns occurring with some frequency include diffuse T-wave inversion, anterior Q waves, and left bundle branch block. ST-segment depression is not common, occurring in fewer than 10% of patients, and its presence should trigger concern for an alternative diagnosis, especially acute coronary syndrome.[19] A normal ECG is observed in approximately 2% of patients[13,14] and sinus rhythm in 90%.[19]

An important element is the frequent evolution of the ECG, typically with progressive T-wave inversion and QT interval lengthening in the course of several days (see **Fig. 2**). In patients with delayed presentation, these changes may be present on admission. This ECG pattern is similar to that observed after successful early reperfusion treatment of acute coronary artery occlusion and is considered a manifestation of electrophysiologic stunning.[33] Rarely, QT prolongation predisposes TTS patients to torsades de pointes ventricular tachycardia (described later). The ECG abnormalities may persist for several weeks, after LV contraction recovery, thus leaving an electrophysiologic footprint of the TTS event.

Cardiac Biomarker Profile

The initial troponin level is elevated in 90% of TTS patients, and troponin release is in a dynamic pattern similar to that of acute myocardial infarction, often leading to a mistaken diagnosis of acute coronary syndrome.[13,14,34] In contrast to acute coronary syndrome, TTS is characterized by substantially lower peak troponin, generally less than 1 ng/mL and less than 3 times baseline troponin value.[19] Higher troponin values warrant consideration for other conditions, such as acute coronary

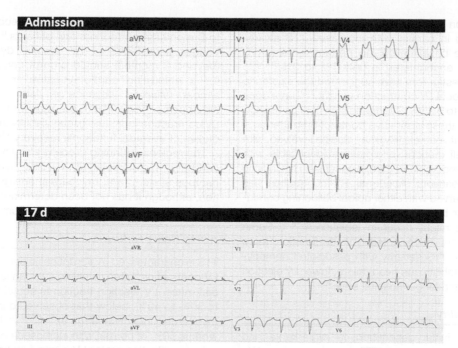

Fig. 2. Evolution of ECG pattern in TTS. Serial 12-lead ECGs in a 56-year-old woman with apical ballooning triggered by gastric hemorrhage demonstrate initial ST-segment elevation with subsequent evolution of T-wave inversion and QTc prolongation. (*Top panel*) Twelve-lead ECG on presentation with ST-segment elevation in leads V2–V6, I, and II and reciprocal ST-segment depression in lead aVR. (*Bottom panel*) ECG 17 days after admission demonstrates diffuse and deep T-wave inversion and QT prolongation (QTc = 531 ms). (*Adapted from* Sharkey SW. Epidemiology and clinical profile of Takotsubo cardiomyopathy. Circ J 2014;78:2123; with permission.)

syndrome or acute myocarditis. As well, creatine kinase release is minimal, generally no greater than 500 U/L.[13,14,19,23] The minor troponin and creatine kinase release despite substantial but reversible LV systolic dysfunction, characteristic of TTS, is consistent with acute myocardial stunning.

Brain natriuretic peptide (BNP) and N-terminal pro-BNP (NT-proBNP) levels may be elevated (median >600 pg/mL and >4000 pg/mL, respectively), often several times greater than those observed with acute coronary syndrome, peaking at 48 hours after presentation, and with elevation for up to 3 months.[19,35] Although BNP and NT-proBNP levels are comparable to those of patients with acute decompensated heart failure, 1 small TTS series reported no association of these biomarkers with either pulmonary congestion or pulmonary capillary wedge pressure, yet a correlation was present with respect to lower LV ejection fraction.[35]

A biomarker with ability to reliably distinguish TTS from ACS would be welcome. Recently, a panel of 4 circulating microRNAs was shown to have 70% specificity for separating acute TTS from ST-segment elevation myocardial infarction (STEMI), thus identifying an area for further study.[36]

Abnormal Contraction Patterns

At least 3 distinct patterns of regional LV contraction failure have been identified, classified as apical ballooning, midballooning, and basal ballooning.[13,14,19,25,37,38] In each, abnormal LV wall motion is generally circumferential and anatomically distinct from that caused by obstructive coronary artery disease.

The apical ballooning pattern is present in 75% to 80% of patients, was the first to be described, and is considered as the original identifying feature from which the name "takotsubo" was derived.[1,13,14,19] As is now known, this name was chosen because the unique end-systolic LV ballooning configuration reminded Japanese physicians of the takotsubo, a submersible pot traditionally used to trap an octopus.

The midventricular ballooning pattern, in which the mid-LV is akinetic, with normal apical and basal contraction, is present in 10% to 20% of patients.[13,14,19,38] In the author and colleagues' Minneapolis Heart Institute experience, the recognition of the midventricular phenotype has expanded in parallel with increased TTS awareness. The basal ballooning pattern remains uncommon, encountered in only 1% to 2%.[13,14,19] Some investigators have suggested the existence of a rare focal LV contraction variant.[19] There does not seem to be any prognostic significance associated with these distinctive contraction patterns.

The right ventricle (RV) may also be involved, with apical wall motion abnormalities identifiable with echocardiographic or cardiovascular MRI (CMR) in 25% of patients. Abnormal RV contraction has been observed with either apical ballooning or midventricular ballooning, with sporadic reports suggesting it might occur in isolation.[15,16,39] Some investigators have noted RV dysfunction as a marker for TTS severity with associated hemodynamic instability and heart failure, lower LV ejection fraction, and longer hospital stay.[40]

Reversibility

From its initial description, a remarkable and intriguing hallmark of TTS has been complete reversibility of myocardial contraction abnormalities and clinical findings. Recovery of LV contraction is gradual, generally occurring over 1 to 2 weeks, although the process may be rapid within

48 hours, or prolonged with delayed recovery of 1 to 2 months reported in a few patients.[8,11,13,14,23] Longer persistence of LV systolic dysfunction (beyond 2 months) should prompt consideration for a coexisting cardiomyopathy. In TTS, the almost universal absence of late gadolinium enhancement on CMR in the region of abnormal LV contraction indicates tissue viability and is predictive of eventual functional recovery.[11,36,41]

The regional stunning process also involves the coronary microcirculation, cardiac sympathetic nervous system, and myocardial energy production, although it has not been determined whether these are primary or secondary phenomena.[42,43]

Acute Heart Failure

TTS is characterized by abrupt cessation of regional LV contraction, often involving substantial myocardial mass. LV ejection fraction is acutely reduced to 30% to 40%, below that observed during acute myocardial infarction (**Fig. 3**).[11,10,19,44] LV stroke work is 50% of normal with increased end-systolic volume reflecting major LV pump function impairment and leading to reduced stroke volume and cardiac output.[44] Simultaneously, LV diastolic function is acutely disturbed with an upward shift in the LV diastolic pressure-volume curve, resulting in

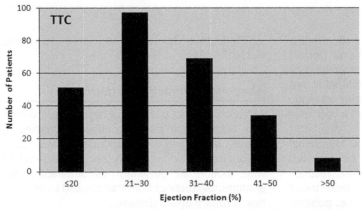

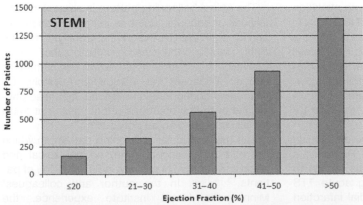

Fig. 3. Distribution of ejection fractions on admission for TTS compared with STEMI. (*Top panel*) TTS in 330 consecutive patients. (*Bottom panel*) STEMI in 3954 consecutive patients. As a group, TTS ejection fraction is significantly lower than STEMI, 32% ± 11% versus 47% ± 14%, respectively, P<.001. (*Adapted from* Sharkey SW. Epidemiology and clinical profile of Takotsubo cardiomyopathy. Circ J 2014;78:2125; with permission.)

substantially elevated LV end-diastolic pressure without significant increase in LV end-diastolic volume.[44] Consequently, TTS patients may experience impressive hemodynamic instability, including profound hypotension (requiring intervention with inotropic drug therapy and/or mechanical circulatory support), pulmonary edema, and cardiogenic shock.[13,14,18,19,23] In the author and colleagues' recent report from the Minneapolis Heart Institute, 15% of 249 TTS patients had unstable hypotension requiring inotropic drugs or IABP, two-thirds of whom had acute pulmonary edema or cardiogenic shock.[18] Similarly, in a contemporary multicenter report involving 1750 TTS patients, cardiogenic shock was observed in 10% and catecholamine use in 12%.[19] Also, an Italian report (227 patients) noted acute heart failure (pulmonary edema and/or oxygen desaturation requiring intervention) in 20% and cardiogenic shock in 8%,[45] whereas a combined German-Austrian TTS registry (324 patients) reported pulmonary edema in 8% and cardiogenic shock in 4%.[17] Taken together, these observations suggest severe hemodynamic instability occurs in 10% to 20% of TTS patients.

The most effective treatment protocol for hypotension or shock associated with TTS has not been established. Hypotension usually responds to intravenous vasopressor drugs, including dopamine, dobutamine, phenylephrine, norepinephrine, and vasopressin. Although these drugs have commonly been used for the treatment of TTS associated hypotension, the use of catecholamine drugs is of concern because these agents have been implicated in the pathophysiology of this condition.[7,13,14,20,21] An analysis from the International Takotsubo Registry demonstrated catecholamine use was an independent predictor of in-hospital death in both men and women.[46] The author and colleagues' Minneapolis Heart Institute cohort has not observed negative clinical consequences directly related to catecholamine administration, and TTS survivors, even when treated with these drugs, experienced complete cardiovascular recovery (including normalization of ejection fraction).[18] Nonetheless, catecholamine drugs should be avoided if possible.[46,47] More profound hemodynamic compromise may require temporary mechanical circulatory support with IABP, LV assist devices, or extracorporeal membrane oxygenation. In certain circumstances, an IABP may cause or aggravate LV outflow tract obstruction leading some investigators to advocate alternative forms of mechanical support as treatment of TTS-associated cardiogenic shock.[48,49] Nonetheless, both LV assist device and extracorporeal membrane oxygenation devices carry nontrivial risks and LV outflow tract obstruction associated with IABP use can be readily assessed with bedside ultrasound.

Beyond reduced ejection fraction, additional factors contribute to hemodynamic instability, including local myocardial edema (present in up to 80% on CMR) leading to impaired LV compliance.[37] Mechanical factors, such as LV outflow tract obstruction and mitral regurgitation, may cause or worsen heart failure.[50] Subaortic obstruction is more common with the apical ballooning pattern, may be provoked or exacerbated by catecholamine drugs used to treat hypotension, and is associated with mitral regurgitation but does not have a negative survival impact.[13,14,50] Intravenous β-blockers have been successful in attenuating LV outflow tract obstruction in hemodynamically unstable TTS patients.[51] After recovery, persistence of mitral valve systolic anterior motion and outflow tract obstruction (with septal hypertrophy) may indicate coexisting hypertrophic cardiomyopathy. Acute reversible mitral valve regurgitation, secondary to systolic anterior mitral valve motion or apical subvalvar tethering, has been reported in 20% of TTS patients and is associated with acute pulmonary edema and cardiogenic shock.[45]

Coronary Artery Disease and Takotsubo Syndrome

Incidental coronary artery disease

Most TTS patients have normal coronary arteries or mild nonobstructive atherosclerosis, although some have reduced contrast flow rate in the epicardial coronary arteries perhaps representing downstream microvascular stunning that usually resolves within several weeks.[32,52] Because the TTS population is older, nonparticipant obstructive coronary artery disease (coronary stenosis remote from the area of abnormal wall motion) may be encountered in an important minority.[14,19,53] This scenario requires careful consideration in choosing appropriate management. For example, it may be inappropriate to perform percutaneous coronary intervention for bystander obstructive coronary disease when the clinical event is TTS.

Acute coronary syndrome mimicking takotsubo syndrome

The apical LV ballooning phenotype is not pathognomonic of TTS, and urgent coronary angiography is necessary to exclude an unstable coronary obstruction that requires revascularization.[13,14] In particular, TTS-like apical ballooning may be the consequence of acute myocardial ischemia in the setting of proximal stenosis involving an LAD, which extends beyond the LV apex to supply the inferior wall (wraparound LAD) (Fig. 4).[54] In uncertain

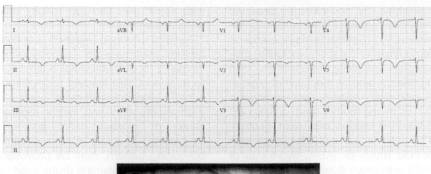

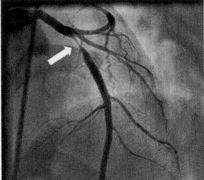

Fig. 4. Acute coronary syndrome due to LAD stenosis initially mimicking TTS. A 48-year-old woman without coronary risk factors presented to the emergency department with acute chest pain after profound emotional distress at work. Initial troponin was elevated, emergent echocardiogram was interpreted as LV apical ballooning consistent with TTS. (*Top panel*) Admission ECG demonstrates prominent T-wave inversion and QTc prolongation to 527 ms. (*Bottom panel*) Left coronary angiogram from right anterior oblique projection demonstrates severe stenosis (*arrow*) in the proximal LAD coronary artery, which was treated with a drug eluting stent. The LAD extends beyond the LV apex to the apical inferior wall (wraparound type).

situations, such as late presentation, suspected coronary embolism, or when coronary angiographic findings are equivocal, CMR is useful because late gadolinium enhancement is rarely evident in TTS but frequently presents in a vascular distribution in patients with ischemic injury from coronary artery disease (**Fig. 5**).[13,14,37]

Acute myocarditis

Acute myocarditis and TTS and share clinical features, including presentation with chest pain, ischemic ECG changes, troponin release, and absent acute coronary artery obstruction. In rare circumstances, acute myocarditis may result in TTS-like regional LV contraction abnormality, in which case it may be challenging to distinguish the 2 conditions.[14,55] In this setting, CMR may be useful because TTS is characterized by myocardial edema in a transmural distribution (T2-weighted imaging) without late gadolinium enhancement.[14,56]

Arrhythmias

Potentially lethal arrhythmias, occurring at presentation or during hospitalization, are part of the clinical spectrum of TTS (in approximately 2% of patients),

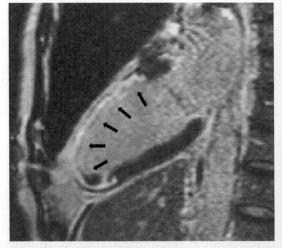

Fig. 5. Delayed gadolinium enhancement (*arrows*) in the distribution of the LAD coronary artery demonstrated by cardiac MRI in the vertical long-axis view. An elderly man was hospitalized with an acute noncardiac illness, an echocardiogram was interpreted as LV apical ballooning consistent with TTS. Coronary angiography demonstrated complete occlusion of wraparound LAD.

including ventricular fibrillation, torsades de pointes ventricular tachycardia, pulseless electrical activity, and asystole.[13,14,18,19,57] In particular, in patients with both TTS and cardiac arrest, it may be uncertain whether TTS should be implicated as the cause or alternatively the consequence of the arrhythmia. The profound physiologic stress of cardiac arrest (and subsequent resuscitation), sometimes with epinephrine administration, might independently trigger a TTS event. Furthermore, catastrophic medical events, such as acute respiratory failure or intracranial hemorrhage, are established TTS triggers and yet can also culminate in cardiac arrest.

Torsades de pointes complicating TTS is observed in the setting of QT interval prolongation greater than 500 ms (**Fig. 6**).[58] Although QT interval lengthening is a common TTS feature, torsades de pointes is rarely reported.[13,14,18,19] Male patients and those with bradycardia and atrial fibrillation seem more susceptible.[59] Because QT lengthening may be progressive and delayed, it is prudent to continue cardiac rhythm monitoring at least until hospital discharge and to avoid drugs that promote QT prolongation.

In the author and colleagues' Minneapolis Heart Institute TTS cohort, cardiac arrest was observed in 4%,[18] which exceeds that reported in the literature and may reflect increased awareness of TTS or the establishment of a local therapeutic hypothermia program, resulting in increased referrals to the hospital (**Fig. 7**). In one-half of these patients, a major noncardiac event (acute respiratory failure from chronic obstructive lung disease or subarachnoid hemorrhage) immediately preceded the cardiac arrest. In the other patients, however, the TTS event itself was the only identifiable substrate for cardiac arrest, and each of these patients received a secondary prevention implantable defibrillator.[18] These observations raise the possibility that TTS itself may be a cause of unexplained sudden death.

Embolic Events

Ventricular thrombi are reported in approximately 5% of TTS patients, may be multiple at sites geographically distinct from those observed in acute myocardial infarction, and can lead to systemic and pulmonary embolic events.[13,14,37,56] CMR has proved more sensitive than 2-D echocardiography for detection of ventricular thrombi in TTS[37,56] and anticoagulation should be considered until LV and RV wall motion has recovered and the risk of thrombus diminished. The efficacy of newer oral anticoagulant drugs (rivaroxaban, dabigatran, and apixaban) as treatment of ventricular thrombi in TTS has not been established.

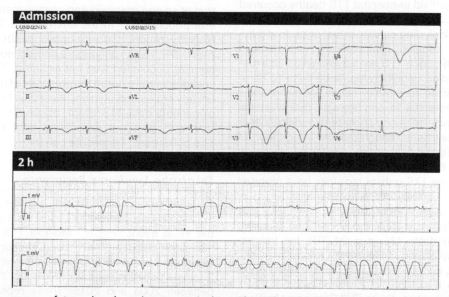

Fig. 6. Occurrence of torsades de pointes ventricular tachycardia in an 84-year-old woman with an apical ballooning TTS event triggered by emotional stress. (*Top panel*) Admission ECG demonstrates sinus bradycardia, prominent T-wave inversion, and QTc prolongation to 549 ms. (*Bottom panel*) Continuous 18 s recording of lead II rhythm strip 2 hours after admission shows sinus bradycardia with paired premature ventricular contractions followed by torsades de pointes ventricular tachycardia, which self-terminated. The patient received a permanent pacemaker for underlying sinus node dysfunction and torsades de pointes resolved with higher heart rate. (*Adapted from* Sharkey SW. Epidemiology and clinical profile of Takotsubo cardiomyopathy. Circ J 2014;78:2124; with permission.)

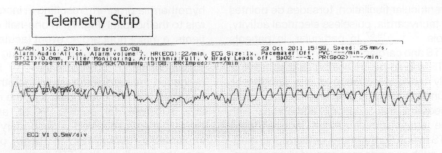

Fig. 7. Ventricular fibrillation on presentation in a 59-year-old man with acute TTS. The patient suffered a panic attack during outpatient withdrawal from chronic narcotic use and presented to the emergency department with chest pain. Ten minutes after arrival, he became unresponsive with ventricular fibrillation on telemetry monitor which responded to a single shock without cardiopulmonary resuscitation or epinephrine. After stabilization, ECG showed ST-segment elevation in anterior leads, and angiography demonstrated normal coronary arteries and midventricular LV ballooning with ejection fraction 30%. The patient completely recovered with follow-up ejection fraction 60% and received an implantable defibrillator before discharge. (*Adapted from* Sharkey SW. Clinical profile of patients with high-risk tako-tsubo cardiomyopathy. Am J Cardiol 2015;116:767; with permission.)

Hospital Mortality

Despite the severity of acute heart failure and LV systolic dysfunction, hospital mortality in TTS is low, with greater than 95% survival and subsequent expectation for complete cardiac recovery. In the author and colleagues' North American Minneapolis experience, hospital survival was 97% (including many with advanced heart failure or cardiogenic shock as complications), with ejection fraction increasing from 32% on admission to 57% at recovery.[18] All in-hospital TTS deaths occurred among patients with a particularly unstable presentation, including cardiac arrest or profound hypotension requiring intravenous vasopressors and/or IABP. Each TTS nonsurvivor also had a major noncardiac condition (eg, subarachnoid hemorrhage, acute respiratory failure, or malignancy) with the potential to compromise clinical status and adversely influence short-term survival. Other investigators have recognized the importance of such coexisting noncardiac conditions having an impact on hospital survival.[16,60–63]

Other large TTS patient registries have reported in-hospital mortality of 2% to 5%, including Germany and Austria (mortality 2%, n = 324), Italy (mortality 3%, n = 227), the US National Inpatient Sample (mortality 4%, n = 24,701), the International Takotsubo Registry (mortality 4%, n = 1750), and an 11-country meta-analysis (mortality 4.5%, n = 2120).[17,19,45,61,62] Hospital mortality is greater in male patients.[18,19] Rare complications resulting in TTS-related death include LV free wall rupture and ventricular septal defect.[13,14]

Posthospital Outcomes

Information regarding long-term survival after a TTS event is limited and unavoidably influenced by the older age of this patient population. The author and colleagues' North American experience has demonstrated higher all-cause mortality for TTS compared with the age-matched and gender-matched general population (**Fig. 8**). Excess mortality occurred predominantly within the first year after the TTS event, usually due to noncardiac conditions, such as malignancy or advanced pulmonary disease.[11,13,18] In contrast, in a smaller North American study, posthospital survival at 4 years did not differ significantly from that of an age-matched and gender-matched general population.[64] In the International Takotsubo Registry report, the any-cause death rate was nearly 6% yearly, although a comparison with the general population was not included.[19] Some investigators have noted the presence of heightened anxiety states and atypical chest pain in a minority of patients post-TTS event, observations consistent with personal experience with the author and colleagues' Minnesota cohort.[14]

Takotsubo Syndrome Recurrence

TTS may reoccur in 5% to 20% of patients appearing as early as 3 weeks or as late as 4 years after the initial event.[11,13,14,64] Multiple TTS events in the same individual have been encountered, for example, the author and colleagues have treated 2 female patients, each with 6 distinct TTS events between 2003 and 2015. These repetitive TTS events were not prevented by standard doses of β-blockers, calcium channel blockers, or angiotensin-converting enzyme inhibitors. Initial and recurrent TTS events have been reported in patients receiving β-blocker therapy, usually administered for coexisting systemic hypertension. In the author and colleagues' cohort,

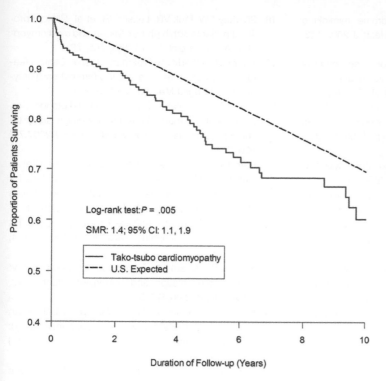

Fig. 8. Kaplan-Meier survival curves for TTS patients versus expected in the general population. Kaplan-Meier survival curves for 249 patients with TTS (*solid red line*) compared with expected in an age-matched and gender-matched US general population (*broken blue line*). SMR, standardized mortality ratio. (*Adapted from* Sharkey SW. Clinical profile of patients with high-risk tako-tsubo cardiomyopathy. Am J Cardiol 2015;116:770; with permission.)

approximately 20% of patients were receiving β-blocker drugs at the time of their initial TTS event and 43% at the time of a second episode.[11] Consistent with this observation, a meta-analysis found no benefit of drug therapy for prevention of TTS recurrence.[65] Inexplicably, in recurrent TTS, the LV ballooning pattern may differ, for example, with apical ballooning during the initial event and midventricular ballooning during the second event.[13,14]

Management

Management of TTS is empiric with no randomized trials to guide treatment of the acute event or prevention of recurrence. Because TTS is a form of acute LV dysfunction with reduced ejection fraction, many patients are treated with β-blockers and/or angiotensin-converting enzyme inhibitors, although there is no evidence these agents promote LV recovery or change outcome in the hospital setting. Retrospective analyses have shown no in-hospital or late survival benefit for β-blocker use in TTS.[19,66] In contrast, 1-year survival was marginally improved with the use of angiotensin-converting enzyme inhibitors or angiotensin-receptor blockers.[19] Until further information becomes available, it has been the author and colleagues' practice to discontinue β-blockers and angiotensin-converting enzyme inhibitors once complete clinical recovery has occurred.

ACKNOWLEDGMENTS

Victoria Pink, RN, CCRC, and Ross Garberich, MS, assisted in the performance of this research and preparation of the article. Dr Barry Maron has provided invaluable expertise and guidance since the inception of the Minneapolis Heart Institute Foundation Tako-Tsubo Research Program.

REFERENCES

1. Dote K, Sato H, Tateishi H, et al. Myocardial stunning due to simultaneous multivessel coronary spasms: a review of 5 cases. J Cardiol 1991;21:203–14 [in Japanese].
2. Sharkey SW, Shear W, Hodges M, et al. Reversible myocardial contraction abnormalities in patients with an acute noncardiac illness. Chest 1998;114:98–105.
3. Sharkey SW, Lesser JR, Zenovich AG, et al. Acute and reversible cardiomyopathy provoked by stress in women from the United States. Circulation 2005;111:472–9.
4. Tsuchihashi K, Ueshima K, Uchida T, et al. Transient left ventricular apical ballooning without coronary artery stenosis: a novel heart syndrome mimicking acute myocardial infarction. Angina Pectoris-Myocardial Infarction Investigations in Japan. J Am Coll Cardiol 2001;38:11–8.
5. Kurisu S, Sato H, Kawagoe T, et al. Tako-tsubo-like left ventricular dysfunction with ST-segment

elevation: a novel cardiac syndrome mimicking acute myocardial infarction. Am Heart J 2002;143: 448–55.

6. Abe Y, Kondo M, Matsuoka R, et al. Assessment of clinical features in transient left ventricular apical ballooning. J Am Coll Cardiol 2003;41:737–42.

7. Wittstein IS, Thiemann DR, Lima JA, et al. Neurohumoral features of myocardial stunning due to sudden emotional stress. N Engl J Med 2005; 352:539–48.

8. Bybee KA, Prasad A. Stress-related cardiomyopathy syndromes. Circulation 2008;118:397–409.

9. Maron BJ, Towbin JA, Thiene G, et al, American Heart Association, Council on Clinical Cardiology, Heart Failure and Transplantation Committee, Quality of Care and Outcomes Research and Functional Genomics and Translational Biology Interdisciplinary Working Groups, Council on Epidemiology and Prevention. Contemporary definitions and classification of the cardiomyopathies. An American Heart Association Scientific Statement from the Council on Clinical Cardiology, Heart Failure and Transplantation Committee; Quality of Care and Outcomes Research and Functional Genomics and Translational Biology Interdisciplinary Working Groups; and Council on Epidemiology and Prevention. Circulation 2006; 113:1807–16.

10. Sharkey SW, Lesser JR, Maron MS, et al. Why not just call it tako-tsubo cardiomyopathy: a discussion of nomenclature. J Am Coll Cardiol 2011;57: 1496–7.

11. Sharkey SW, Windenburg DC, Lesser JR, et al. Natural history and expansive clinical profile of stress (tako-tsubo) cardiomyopathy. J Am Coll Cardiol 2010;55:333–41.

12. Bossone E, Erbel R. The "takotsubo syndrome": from legend to science. Heart Failure Clin 2013;9:xiii–xv.

13. Sharkey SW, Maron BJ. Epidemiology and clinical profile of Takotsubo cardiomyopathy. Circ J 2014; 78:2119–28.

14. Lyon AR, Bossone E, Schneider B, et al. Current state of knowledge on Takotsubo syndrome: a position statement from the taskforce on takotsubo syndrome of the heart failure association of the European Society of Cardiology. Eur J Heart Fail 2015;18(1):8–27.

15. Deshmukh A, Kumar G, Pant S, et al. Prevalence of Takotsubo cardiomyopathy in the United States. Am Heart J 2012;164:66–71.

16. Murugiah K, Wang Y, Desai NR, et al. Trends in Short- and Long-Term Outcomes for Takotsubo Cardiomyopathy Among Medicare Fee-for-Service Beneficiaries, 2007 to 2012. JACC Heart Fail 2016;4: 197–205.

17. Schneider B, Athanasiadis A, Sechtem U. Gender-related differences in takotsubo cardiomyopathy. Heart Failure Clin 2013;9:137–46, vii.

18. Sharkey SW, Pink VR, Lesser JR, et al. Clinical profile of patients with high-risk Tako-tsubo cardiomyopathy. Am J Cardiol 2015;116(5):765–72.

19. Templin C, Ghadri JR, Diekmann J, et al. Clinical features and outcomes of takotsubo (stress) cardiomyopathy. N Engl J Med 2015;373:929–38.

20. Kawai S, Kitabatake A, Tomoike H, Takotsubo Cardiomyopathy Group. Guidelines for diagnosis of takotsubo (ampulla) cardiomyopathy. Circ J 2007;71: 990–2.

21. Parodi G, Citro R, Bellandi B, et al, Tako-tsubo Italian Network (TIN). Revised clinical diagnostic criteria for Tako-tsubo syndrome: the Tako-tsubo Italian Network proposal. Int J Cardiol 2014;172:282–3.

22. Sharkey SW. What medicare knows about the Takotsubo cardiomyopathy. JACC Heart Fail 2016;4: 206–7.

23. Kurisu S, Kihara Y. Tako-tsubo cardiomyopathy: Clinical presentation and underlying mechanism. J Cardiol 2012;60:429–37.

24. Prasad A, Lerman A, Rihal CS. Apical ballooning syndrome (Tako-Tsubo or stress cardiomyopathy): a mimic of acute myocardial infarction. Am Heart J 2008;155:408–17.

25. Park JH, Kang SJ, Song JK, et al. Left ventricular apical ballooning due to severe physical stress in patients admitted to the medical ICU. Chest 2005; 128:296–302.

26. Haghi D, Fluechter S, Suselbeck T, et al. Takotsubo cardiomyopathy (acute left ventricular apical ballooning syndrome) occurring in the intensive care unit. Intensive Care Med 2006;32:1069–74.

27. Summers MR, Prasad A. Takotsubo cardiomyopathy: definition and clinical profile. Heart Failure Clin 2013;9:111–22, vii.

28. Agarwal V, Kant G, Hans N, et al. Takotsubo-like cardiomyopathy in pheochromocytoma. Int J Cardiol 2011;153:241–8.

29. Sharkey SW, McAllister N, Dassenko D, et al. Evidence that high catecholamine levels produced by pheochromocytoma may be responsible for Takotsubo cardiomyopathy. Am J Cardiol 2015;115: 1615–8.

30. Abraham J, Mudd JO, Kapur N, et al. Stress cardiomyopathy after intravenous administration of catecholamines and beta-receptor agonists. J Am Coll Cardiol 2009;53:1320–5.

31. Johnson NP, Chavez JF, Mosley WJ 2nd, et al. Performance of electrocardiographic criteria to differentiate Takotsubo cardiomyopathy from acute anterior ST elevation myocardial infarction. Int J Cardiol 2013;164:345–8.

32. Sharkey SW, Lesser JR, Menon M, et al. Spectrum and significance of electrocardiographic patterns, troponin levels, and thrombolysis in myocardial infarction frame count in patients with stress (tako-tsubo) cardiomyopathy and comparison to those in

patients with ST-elevation anterior wall myocardial infarction. Am J Cardiol 2008;101:1723–8.

33. Kosuge M, Ebina T, Hibi K, et al. Differences in negative T waves between takotsubo cardiomyopathy and reperfused anterior acute myocardial infarction. Circ J 2012;76:462–8.

34. Fröhlich GM, Schoch B, Schmid F, et al. Takotsubo cardiomyopathy has a unique cardiac biomarker profile: NT-proBNP/myoglobin and NT-proBNP/troponin T ratios for the differential diagnosis of acute coronary syndromes and stress induced cardiomyopathy. Int J Cardiol 2012;154: 328–32.

35. Nguyen TH, Neil CJ, Sverdlov AL, et al. N-terminal pro-brain natriuretic protein levels in takotsubo cardiomyopathy. Am J Cardiol 2011;108: 1316–21.

36. Jaguszewski M, Osipova J, Ghadri JR, et al. A signature of circulating microRNAs differentiates takotsubo cardiomyopathy from acute myocardial infarction. Eur Heart J 2014;35:999–1006.

37. Eitel I, von Knobelsdorff-Brenkenhoff F, Bernhardt P, et al. Clinical characteristics and cardiovascular magnetic resonance findings in stress (takotsubo) cardiomyopathy. JAMA 2011;306:277–86.

38. Hurst RT, Askew JW, Reuss CS, et al. Transient mid-ventricular ballooning syndrome: a new variant. J Am Coll Cardiol 2006;48:579–83.

39. Stahl B. Isolated right ventricular ballooning. Eur Heart J 2011;32:1821.

40. Elesber AA, Prasad A, Bybee KA, et al. Transient cardiac apical ballooning syndrome: prevalence and clinical implications of right ventricular involvement. J Am Coll Cardiol 2006;47:1082–3.

41. Mitchell JH, Hadden TB, Wilson JM, et al. Clinical features and usefulness of cardiac magnetic resonance imaging in assessing myocardial viability and prognosis in takotsubo cardiomyopathy (transient left ventricular apical ballooning syndrome). Am J Cardiol 2007;100:296–301.

42. Alexanderson E. Transient perfusion and motion abnormalities in takotsubo cardiomyopathy. J Nucl Cardiol 2007;14:129–33.

43. Sato A, Aonuma K, Nozato T, et al. Stunned myocardium in transient left ventricular apical ballooning: a serial study of dual i-123 bmipp and tl-201 spect. J Nucl Cardiol 2008;15:671–9.

44. Medeiros K, O'Connor MJ, Baicu CF, et al. Systolic and diastolic mechanics in stress cardiomyopathy. Circulation 2014;129:1659–67.

45. Citro R, Rigo F, D'Andrea A, et al. Echocardiographic correlates of acute heart failure, cardiogenic shock, and in-hospital mortality in tako-tsubo cardiomyopathy. JACC Cardiovasc Imaging 2014;7:119–29.

46. Templin C, Ghadri JR, Napp LC. Takotsubo (stress) cardiomyopathy. N Engl J Med 2015;373:2689–91.

47. Padayachee L. Levosimendan: The inotrope of choice in cardiogenic shock secondary to takotsubo cardiomyopathy? Heart Lung Circ 2007;16: S65–70.

48. Good CW, Hubbard CR, Harrison TA, et al. Echocardiographic guidance in treatment of cardiogenic shock complicating transient left ventricular apical ballooning syndrome. JACC Cardiovasc Imaging 2009;2:372–4.

49. Rashed A, Won S, Saad M, et al. Use of the Impella 2.5 left ventricular assist device in a patient with cardiogenic shock secondary to takotsubo cardiomyopathy. BMJ Case Rep 2015;2015.

50. De Backer O, Debonnaire P, Gevaert S, et al. Prevalence, associated factors and management implications of left ventricular outflow tract obstruction in takotsubo cardiomyopathy: a two-year, two-center experience. BMC Cardiovasc Disord 2014; 14:147.

51. Angue M, Soubirou L, Vandroux D, et al. Beneficial effects of intravenous beta-blockers in Tako-Tsubo syndrome with dynamic left ventricular outflow tract obstruction and severe haemodynamic impairment. Int J Cardiol 2014;177:e56–7.

52. Bybee KA, Prasad A, Barsness GW, et al. Clinical characteristics and thrombolysis in myocardial infarction frame counts in women with transient left ventricular apical ballooning syndrome. Am J Cardiol 2004;94:343–6.

53. Kurisu S. Prevalence of incidental coronary artery disease in tako-tsubo cardiomyopathy. Coron Artery Dis 2009;20:214–8.

54. Chao T, Lindsay J, Collins S, et al. Can acute occlusion of the left anterior descending coronary artery produce a typical "takotsubo" left ventricular contraction pattern? Am J Cardiol 2009;104: 202–4.

55. Caforio AL, Tona F, Vinci A, et al. Acute biopsy-proven lymphocytic myocarditis mimicking Takotsubo cardiomyopathy. Eur J Heart Fail 2009;11: 428–31.

56. Athanasiadis A, Schneider B, Sechtem U. Role of cardiovascular magnetic resonance in takotsubo cardiomyopathy. Heart Failure Clin 2013;9: 167–76, viii.

57. Syed FF, Asirvatham SJ, Francis J. Arrhythmia occurrence with takotsubo cardiomyopathy: a literature review. Europace 2011;13:780–8.

58. Madias C, Fitzgibbons TP, Alsheikh-Ali AA, et al. Acquired long QT syndrome from stress cardiomyopathy is associated with ventricular arrhythmias and torsades de pointes. Heart Rhythm 2011;8: 555–61.

59. Samuelov-Kinori L, Kinori M, Kogan Y, et al. Takotsubo cardiomyopathy and QT interval prolongation: who are the patients at risk for torsades de pointes? J Electrocardiol 2009;42:353–7.

60. Joe BH, Jo U, Kim HS, et al. APACHE II score, rather than cardiac function, may predict poor prognosis in patients with stress-induced cardiomyopathy. J Korean Med Sci 2012;27:52–7.

61. Brinjikji W, El-Sayed AM, Salka S. In-hospital mortality among patients with takotsubo cardiomyopathy: A study of the National Inpatient Sample 2008 to 2009. Am Heart J 2012;164:215–21.

62. Singh K, Carson K, Shah R, et al. Meta-Analysis of clinical correlates of acute mortality in takotsubo cardiomyopathy. Am J Cardiol 2014;113:1420–8.

63. Pelliccia F, Parodi G, Greco C, et al. Comorbidities frequency in Takotsubo syndrome: an international collaborative systematic review including 1109 patients. Am J Med 2015;128:654.e11-9.

64. Elesber AA, Prasad A, Lennon RJ, et al. Four-year recurrence rate and prognosis of the apical ballooning syndrome. J Am Coll Cardiol 2007;50:448–52.

65. Santoro F, Ieva R, Musaico F, et al. Lack of efficacy of drug therapy in preventing takotsubo cardiomyopathy recurrence: a meta-analysis. Clin Cardiol 2014;37:434–9.

66. Isogai T, Matsui H, Tanaka H, et al. Early β-blocker use and in-hospital mortality in patients with Takotsubo cardiomyopathy. Heart 2016. http://dx.doi.org/10.1136/heartjnl-2015-308712.

Influence of Age and Gender in Takotsubo Syndrome

Birke Schneider, MD[a],*, Udo Sechtem, MD[b]

KEYWORDS

- Takotsubo syndrome • Gender-related difference • Emotional stress • Physical stress
- QT prolongation • Ventricular tachycardia • Resuscitation • Apical ballooning syndrome

KEY POINTS

- There is a marked gender preference in Takotsubo syndrome (TTS), 90% of cases are females (mean age, 62 to 76 years). However, younger individuals and even children may also develop TTS.
- In contrast with studies with a "true" acute coronary syndrome, mean age, prehospital delay, and clinical symptoms are similar in male and female patients.
- Physical stress as a triggering event is more frequent in male patients, whereas emotional stress or no identifiable trigger are more prevalent in women.
- The elevation of cardiac markers is higher in males, which may be related to physical stress as a trigger directly before the onset of TTS in men.
- Further studies are necessary to clarify the pathogenetic background and develop strategies against this potentially life-threatening disease.

INTRODUCTION

Many features of Takotsubo syndrome (TTS) have puzzled doctors trying to understand the pathophysiology of this entity, which was first described in Japan in 1990.[1] One of these features is the overwhelming preponderance of women. Moreover, this is a disease mainly of elderly postmenopausal women; younger women seem to be only occasionally affected. In all studies reported so far, there is this marked gender discrepancy, although small numbers of males have also been described.[1–13]

This review summarizes the current knowledge on the epidemiology and clinical presentation of TTS, focusing on age and gender.

PATHOPHYSIOLOGIC BACKGROUND

The precise pathophysiology of TTS and its gender preference are still not well-understood. As possible underlying mechanisms, transient multivessel coronary artery spasm,[1,14,15] coronary microvascular dysfunction,[16–20] and obstruction of the left ventricular (LV) outflow tract[4,7,8,21,22] owing to a septal bulge have been proposed, all of which are more prevalent in women. The most widely accepted hypothesis suggests that TTS is caused by an excessive release of catecholamines after exposure to emotional or physical stress,[8,21,23] resulting in catecholamine-induced myocardial stunning.[24] Similar regional wall motion abnormalities have been observed in patients with high catecholamine levels owing to pheochromocytoma.[25,26] The reason why females should respond more intensely to such stimuli is unknown, but the greater prevalence of microvascular abnormalities in females may play an important role. Estrogen may have a protective role on the cardiovascular system of postmenopausal females by attenuating catecholamine and glucocorticoid response to mental stress

[a] Medizinische Klinik II, Sana Kliniken Lübeck, Kronsforder Allee 71 – 73, Lübeck D-23560, Germany;
[b] Abteilung für Kardiologie, Robert-Bosch-Krankenhaus, Auerbachstrasse 110, Stuttgart D-70376, Germany
* Corresponding author.
E-mail address: birke.schneider@sana.de

Heart Failure Clin 12 (2016) 521–530
http://dx.doi.org/10.1016/j.hfc.2016.06.001
1551-7136/16/$ – see front matter © 2016 Elsevier Inc. All rights reserved.

and by improving norepinephrine-induced vaso-constriction,[27,28] although there are no clinical data confirming a protective effect of hormone replacement therapy against the occurrence of TTS.[29] The reduction of estrogen levels after menopause may predispose elderly women to develop TTS[30–32] and can in part explain the striking female predominance of this syndrome.

EPIDEMIOLOGY AND DEMOGRAPHICS

The true incidence of TTS is unknown. There are most likely minor forms of this syndrome that are not severe enough to result in hospital admission; however, there may also be severe forms of TTS leading to death before the patient can reach the hospital. Approximately 1% to 3% of all patients with a suspected acute coronary syndrome (ACS) undergoing coronary angiography are diagnosed with TTS.[16,33–37] There is a gender-specific prevalence that is higher in women, ranging from 6% to 9.8%, whereas the prevalence of TTS among male patients with an ACS is less than 0.5%.[35–37] It is estimated that there are approximately 50,000 to 100,000 TTS cases per annum in the United States, with similar estimated numbers in Europe.[38,39]

The majority (90%) of individuals with TTS are elderly postmenopausal women with a mean age of 67 years.[3,11–13,38–41] The distribution of females and males in major studies is shown in **Table 1**. In case series from Western countries, less than 11% of the patients are men. The number of men, however, seems to be higher in prospective studies from Asia ranging from 13% to 35%.[3,42,43]

AGE

Although the average age of patients with TTS is around 65 years, approximately 10% of the patients are less than 50 years of age,[3,13] and even young individuals as well as children of both genders may be affected. Several studies look into the gender-specific age distribution of patients with TTS.[13,40,43–45] In most reports, TTS occurs in both sexes at a similar age. However, females were found to be significantly older in 2 studies.[13,43] This may be explained by the fact that up to 21% of the male patients included into these registries also had coronary artery disease where male patients are known to be consistently 7 to 9 years younger than females.[46,47]

Older Age

Elderly patients (≥75 years of age) are considered to be at a greater risk of developing TTS and related major complications (**Box 1**). They experience more in-hospital composite adverse events and a higher in-hospital mortality (6.3% vs 2.8%). In this patient population, a higher frequency of acute heart failure and a longer time to recovery of LV function has also been reported. In addition, right ventricular involvement is more frequently seen in elderly patients as well as thrombus formation and a higher rate of stroke.[13,48–50]

Younger Age

There are some case reports of younger females experiencing TTS in the context of normal pregnancy,[51] after miscarriage, and after labor or delivery.[52–55] The postpartum period may be at

---

Table 1
Age and gender in Takotsubo syndrome

Author, Year	Country	No. of Patients	Age (y)	Female (%)	Male (%)
Tsuchihashi et al,[3] 2001	Japan	88	67 ± 13	86	14
Song et al,[42] 2012	Korea	137	59 ± 12	74	26
Murakami et al,[43] 2015	Japan	368	76 ± 9	77	23
Elesber et al,[9] 2007	USA	100	66 ± 13	95	5
Regnante et al, 2009[79]	USA	70	67 ± 11	95	5
Sharkey et al,[40] 2010	USA	136	68 ± 13	96	4
Schneider et al,[11] 2010	Germany	324	68 ± 12	91	9
Parodi et al,[37] 2011	Italy	116	73 ± 10	91	9
Eitel et al,[12] 2011	Germany	256	69 ± 12	89	11
Citro et al,[48] 2012	Italy	190	66 ± 11	92	8
Chong et al, 2012[80]	Australia	80	68 ± 12	97	3
Schultz et al, 2012[81]	Sweden	115	64 ± 11	86	14
Templin et al,[13] 2015	Europe, USA	1750	67 ± 13	90	10

<table>
<tr><td>

Box 1
Takotsubo syndrome in patients ≥ 75 years

Old age (≥75 years) in Takotsubo syndrome is associated with

- More in-hospital composite adverse events
- Higher in-hospital mortality
- Higher frequency of acute heart failure
- More thrombus formation in the left ventricle
- Higher rate of stroke
- More frequently right ventricular involvement
- Longer time to recovery of left ventricular function

</td></tr>
</table>

increased risk for TTS development owing to the abrupt depletion of estrogen levels after expulsion of the placenta. In addition, and in particular after cesarean delivery, TTS may be precipitated by either an intense emotional and/or physical stress of the simultaneous administration of catecholamines, which are often used to stimulate uterine contraction.[52] There are several features distinguishing postpartum TTS from peripartum cardiomyopathy (PPCM). TTS symptoms arise rather suddenly with rapid worsening of the clinical condition, whereas the onset of PPCM is insidious and signs of heart failure predominate. LV function in PPCM mostly is diffusely reduced, whereas TTS exhibits the typical apical ballooning or its variant forms. Whereas recovery in TTS is normally within a few weeks, recovery of LV function may take several months in PPCM. This corresponds with a usually better prognosis in TTS than in PPCM.[52] However, a recent report using cardiac magnetic resonance imaging disclosed regional wall motion abnormalities and right ventricular involvement in 88% and 35% of the patients, respectively. In many of these cases PPCM resembled an "inverted Takotsubo-like cardiomyopathy," but could be distinguished from TTS by the presence of subepicardial or midwall late gadolinium enhancement.[56]

TTS may also occur in young adults in situations after amphetamine abuse,[57] application of catecholamines,[58] and in young men with cerebral disorders.[59] In all of these cases, a basal (or "inverted") pattern of LV dysfunction was found. Several reports confirm that this unusual end-systolic configuration of the LV (**Fig. 1**) is more frequently found in younger TTS patients.[60–62] Another group of young adults in whom TTS may occur are those with anorexia nervosa. TTS in these cases is most likely triggered by stress resulting from hypoglycemia.[63]

Takotsubo Syndrome in Children

Although TTS is mostly diagnosed in elderly patients, newborns and children with this condition have also been described. The youngest individual affected by TTS was 2 days old and the onset of acute heart failure was triggered by fetal stress and hypoxemia.[64] Another group of children suffering from TTS are those undergoing surgery or in the context of morphine withdrawal.[64–68] Overall, triggering factors, presentation, clinical course, electrocardiography (ECG), and echocardiographic findings are similar in children and adults. TTS in children may be an underappreciated entity owing to the fact that pediatric cardiologists may not be fully aware of the existence of this syndrome in minors. Thus, TTS is frequently interpreted as myocarditis or dilated cardiomyopathy,[64] but this disease entity has to be included in the differential diagnosis of acute heart failure

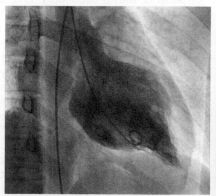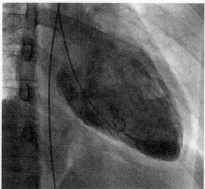

Fig. 1. Left ventricular angiogram at end-systole (*left*) and end-diastole (*right*) in a 21-year-old male with appendicitis, anxiety, and chest pain demonstrating a basal Takotsubo pattern. (*From* Marti V, Carreras F, Pujadas S, et al. Transient left ventricular basal ballooning-"inverted" Takotsubo. Clin Cardiol 2009;32(7):E20; with permission.)

syndromes in all age groups. A unifying patho-physiologic theory explaining why some children react to severe forms of emotional or physical stress by developing TTS does not yet exist.

GENDER-RELATED DIFFERENCES IN TAKOTSUBO SYNDROME

One still poorly understood aspect of TTS is the marked gender discrepancy. Besides pathophysiologic differences in the cardiovascular system, such as the higher prevalence of microvascular abnormalities[69–71] predisposing females to develop TTS, it is currently unclear whether under-diagnosis or misdiagnosis may contribute to the apparent lower prevalence of TTS in men. The diagnosis of TTS depends to some degree on clinically considering the syndrome as a differential diagnosis. If coronary angiography and LV angiography in men show diffuse coronary artery disease and regional LV dysfunction, this is usually interpreted as the result of plaque rupture or coronary embolization. However, searching for details in the history and studying serial ECGs could potentially reveal more cases of TTS also in male patients.[45]

Another reason for underestimating the prevalence of TTS in males could be that males die more often suddenly in the early phase of TTS and the diagnosis cannot be established because the typical course of this syndrome with rapid resolution of the wall abnormality cannot be documented. The fact that males arrived at the hospital more often after resuscitation[45] indicates a greater electrical vulnerability in the early phase of TTS.[66,72] To our knowledge, no comparison of gender-specific reactions to various types of physical or emotional stress in animal models has been reported so far.

Triggering Events

In the majority of patients (70%–80%) with TTS, a triggering event can be identified. Emotional and physical stress events are equally distributed and present in 30% to 40% of the patients, respectively.[45,73] However, these data depend to a great deal on the precision of clinical history taking, which may vary in large registries. Moreover, it may be difficult to differentiate between physical and emotional stressors because factors such as asthma attacks (physical stressor) may lead to panic reactions (emotional stressor). In some registries, such indeterminate histories were summarized in a separate group and both stressor types were assumed to be present.[45]

In most studies looking at gender differences in TTS, physical stress (most commonly acute noncardiac illness or surgical/diagnostic procedures) was significantly more frequent in male patients with TTS, and emotional stress or no identifiable trigger were more prevalent in women.[13,43,45] These findings are in accordance with smaller studies where physical stress was also found to be the predominant stressor in men.[29,40,44]

Prehospital Delay

Data reporting about time intervals from symptom onset to hospital admission vary from study to study, ranging from a median of 2 hours (interquartile range, 1–5) and up to 10 ± 16 hours.[7,8,11,74] In a study specifically evaluating gender differences in TTS, prehospital delay was 7.5 ± 6.9 hours and comparable in women and men.[45] In contrast, patients with an ACS enrolled in a similar hospital setting had a shorter mean prehospital delay, which was significantly longer in female than in male patients (median of 6.2 vs 5.1 hours for non–ST-elevation myocardial infarction and a median of 3.3 vs 2.5 hours for ST-elevation myocardial infarction; both $P<.001$).[46,75] These data imply that symptoms associated with TTS may be less severe than in ACS, have a more insidious onset and are taken less seriously because patients attribute the symptoms mainly to the triggering event preceding TTS onset.[45]

Symptoms

The most common presenting symptoms in TTS are chest pain and dyspnea, which have been reported in 70% and 20% of the patients, respectively.[73] However, initial presentation with syncope, cardiogenic shock, and ventricular fibrillation has also been observed.[3,7,8,11,40,66,74] In addition, nonspecific symptoms such as general weakness[23] or nausea and vomiting may occur. In patients with a secondary TTS, symptoms of the underlying disease may prevail.[39]

When comparing female and male patients with TTS, chest pain was reported more frequently in women; dyspnea, syncope, and no or other symptoms occurred with similar frequency in male and female patients.[13,43,45] Significantly more male patients were admitted after out-of-hospital cardiac arrest and/or in cardiogenic shock and unable to report specific cardiac symptoms.[45] Thus, TTS may be another important cause of cardiac arrest especially in males and should be added to the list of diseases potentially leading to sudden cardiac death. This is substantiated by a study comprising 91 Japanese patients (85% male) who underwent autopsy after sudden cardiac death. In that study, acute cardiac dysfunction related to stress was found to be the most likely cause of death in 19.8%.[76]

Electrocardiogram

The most frequently encountered finding on the admission ECG is ST-segment elevation in the precordial leads which has been documented in 40% to 90% of the patients.[13,45,73] Over the next days, ST-segment elevation resolves and widespread deep T-wave inversion develops. The corrected QT interval is prolonged, and transient Q-waves may be present on admission.[39]

In Japanese studies directly comparing ECG changes in male and female patients with TTS,[43,44] ST-segment elevation on the admission ECG was found less frequently in men and was explained by a presumably later diagnosis of TTS in males. This is in contrast with other studies either reporting no significant difference[13,29] and a large European registry[45] where there was a trend toward a higher number of male patients with ST-segment elevation (96% vs 85%; $P = .09$) despite a similar prehospital delay. Other ECG parameters in this study (heart rate, T-wave inversion, or Q-wave) evaluated during the first 3 days after symptom onset were not different among females and males. In both genders, there is a prolongation of the QTc interval[29,45] with a maximum on the second day after symptom onset.[45] The QTc interval was found to be longer in women than in men only on the day of symptom onset, however, during the following 2 days there was no significant difference between both sexes.[45] Because women normally have a longer QTc interval than men,[77] there may be a disproportionate QTc prolongation in male patients during the acute course of TTS predisposing them to ventricular arrhythmias. Accordingly, in a metaanalysis on QT interval prolongation in TTS patients, a higher prevalence of male sex with torsades de pointes tachycardia has been reported.[72] Men with a prolonged QTc interval are particularly at risk for malignant ventricular arrhythmias (**Fig. 2**); therefore, monitoring for at least 3 days after symptom onset has been suggested.[45]

Laboratory Findings

Elevation of creatine kinase has been reported in 50% to 60% of the patients. Cardiac troponin (measured by conventional assays) was found to be elevated in greater than 90% of TTS patients.[39] In general, the increase of cardiac markers is less than in patients with acute myocardial infarction[39] and seems to be disproportionately low as compared with the extent of LV dysfunction.

Creatine kinase and troponin were found to be higher in male than in female patients.[43,45] The higher level of these cardiac markers in male patients may in part be related to physical stress directly before the onset of TTS.

Plasma brain natriuretic peptide is invariably elevated in patients with TTS,[39] and elevation of catecholamines has been observed in many patients.[39] Higher maximum brain natriuretic peptide levels were seen in female patients, although their LV ejection fraction was higher than in males.[13,29]

Angiographic Findings

Coronary angiography in patients with TTS typically shows absence of culprit atherosclerotic

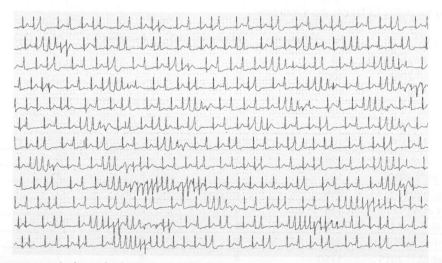

Fig. 2. Malignant ventricular arrhythmias in a male patient with Takotsubo syndrome on day 2 after symptom onset. There is marked prolongation of the QTc interval (628 ms), resulting in torsades de pointes tachycardia.

coronary artery disease including acute plaque rupture, thrombus formation, and coronary dissection or other pathologic conditions to explain the pattern of temporary LV dysfunction observed. Left ventriculography reveals regional wall motion abnormalities usually extending beyond a single epicardial vascular distribution and typically shows a circumferential dysfunction of the ventricular segments involved.[39]

Time from symptom onset to angiography was similar in female and male patients. Gender differences in LV ejection fraction are small but values tend to be greater in females.[29,43,45] This difference was significant, however, in only 1 registry.[13] The frequency of an apical versus midventricular ballooning pattern was similar in female and male patients.[13,45] As expected, the extent of accompanying coronary artery disease was more pronounced in males.[13,29,45]

Complications

A variety of complications have been reported in the course of the disease, such as malignant arrhythmias, cardiogenic shock, pulmonary edema, intraventricular pressure gradients sometimes associated with acute mitral regurgitation, right ventricular involvement with pleural effusions, intraventricular thrombi resulting in stroke and arterial embolism, pericardial effusion, or ventricular wall rupture. In-hospital mortality was observed in 2% to 5% of TTS patients.[39]

Complications during hospitalization occur in a high proportion (20%–53%) of both female and male patients.[13,43,45] In 1 study, pulmonary edema was seen more frequently in women than in men[45]; however, a heart failure Killip class of III or greater and the need for mechanical ventilation in other studies was more frequently observed in men.[13,29,45] The frequency of right ventricular involvement, occurrence of intraventricular pressure gradients, arrhythmias, and need for resuscitation or development of cardiogenic shock in men and women varies between studies; a clear gender difference was not consistently observed.

Mortality was similar for men and women in some studies (**Table 2**), but 1 large registry saw a significantly higher mortality in men. However, this study also had the greatest proportion of men with concomitant coronary artery disease included.[13] Two studies looking at patients identified by the *International Classification of Disease* code for TTS also found a higher mortality in men than in women.[50,78] Again, the higher mortality in men in these 2 studies could have been potentially caused by erroneous classification of male CAD patients as TTS patients in populations with a large proportion of patients with previous diagnoses of atherosclerotic disease or secondary TTS.[50]

Recurrence

Five-year recurrence rates of 5% to 22% after an initial TTS have been reported, with the second episode occurring 3 months to 10 years after the first.[39] One study[29] found a higher recurrence rate in younger female patients, but most studies report no difference between the sexes.[13,45] Hormone replacement therapy does not exclude the risk for developing TTS.[29]

Table 2
Thirty-day mortality in Takotsubo syndrome

Author, Year	No. of Patients	Mortality (%)	Female (%)	Male (%)	P Value
Tsuchihashi et al,[3] 2001	88	1	—	—	—
Elesber et al,[9] 2007	100	2	—	—	—
Song et al,[42] 2012	137	0	—	—	—
Sharkey et al,[40] 2010	136	2	—	—	—
Parodi et al,[37] 2011	116	2	—	—	—
Citro et al,[48] 2012	190	3	—	—	—
Schneider et al,[11] 2010	324	2	2	0	ns
Kurisu et al,[44] 2010	102	7	6	15	ns
Eitel et al,[12] 2011	256	2	1	3	ns
Schultz et al, 2012[81]	115	6	6	7	ns
Singh et al,[78] 2014	2120	4	4	8	<.02
Murakami et al,[43] 2015	368	6	5	9	ns
Templin et al,[13] 2015	1750	4	4	7	.025

Abbreviation: ns, not significant.

SUMMARY

TTS occurs predominantly in elderly females. Males are affected in about 10% of the patients in Western countries with a similar clinical profile. According to some large registries, there are no consistent differences between men and women with respect to age, frequency of symptoms at presentation, prehospital delay, or clinical course. Mortality has been reported to be higher in males in some large retrospective registries but this could be owing to inadvertent inclusion of more male patients with coronary artery disease. The QTc interval may be disproportionately prolonged in male patients in the days after admission predisposing them to malignant ventricular arrhythmias. The higher level of cardiac markers found in male patients with TTS may in part be related to the greater frequency of physical stress directly before the onset of TTS in men. TTS needs to be further investigated at the clinical and experimental level in men and women separately to explain the pathophysiology of this disease resulting in a marked gender difference. Understanding the pathogenetic background may in the end lead to the development of preventive and therapeutic means against this life-threatening disease.

REFERENCES

1. Sato H, Tateishi H, Uchida T, et al. Takotsubo like left ventricular dysfunction due to multivessel coronary spasm. In: Kodama K, Haze K, Hon M, editors. Clinical aspect of myocardial injury: from ischemia to heart failure. Tokyo: Kagakuhyouronsya Publishing Co; 1990. p. 56–64 [in Japanese].
2. Kawai S, Suzuki H, Yamaguchi H, et al. Ampulla cardiomyopathy ("Takotusbo" Cardiomyopathy). Reversible left ventricular dysfunction with ST segment elevation. Jpn Circ J 2000;64:156–9.
3. Tsuchihashi K, Ueshima K, Uchida T, et al. Transient left ventricular apical ballooning without coronary artery stenosis: a novel heart syndrome mimicking acute myocardial infarction. J Am Coll Cardiol 2001;38:11–8.
4. Kurisu S, Sato H, Kawagoe T, et al. Tako-tsubo like left ventricular dysfunction with ST-segment elevation: a novel cardiac syndrome mimicking acute myocardial infarction. Am Heart J 2002;143:448–55.
5. Abe Y, Kondo M, Matsuoka R, et al. Assessment of clinical features in transient left ventricular apical ballooning. J Am Coll Cardiol 2003;41:737–42.
6. Desmet WJ, Adriaenssens BF, Dens JA. Apical ballooning of the left ventricle: first series in white patients. Heart 2003;89:1027–31.
7. Sharkey SW, Lesser JR, Zenovich AG, et al. Acute and reversible cardiomyopathy provoked by stress in women from the United States. Circulation 2005; 111:472–9.
8. Wittstein IS, Thiemann DR, Lima JA, et al. Neurohumoral features of myocardial stunning due to sudden emotional stress. N Engl J Med 2005;352: 539–48.
9. Elesber AA, Prasad A, Lennon RJ, et al. Four-year recurrence rate and prognosis of the apical ballooning syndrome. J Am Coll Cardiol 2007;50: 448–52.
10. Parodi G, Del Pace S, Salvadori C, et al. Tuscany Registry of Tako-Tsubo Cardiomyopathy. Left ventricular apical ballooning syndrome as a novel cause of acute mitral regurgitation. J Am Coll Cardiol 2007; 50:647–9.
11. Schneider B, Athanasiadis A, Schwab J, et al. Clinical spectrum of Takotsubo cardiomyopathy in Germany: results of the Takotsubo registry of the Arbeitsgemeinschaft Leitende Kardiologische Krankenhausärzte (ALKK). Dtsch Med Wochenschr 2010;135:1908–13.
12. Eitel I, von Knobelsdorff-Brenkenhoff F, Bernhardt P, et al. Clinical characteristics and cardiovascular magnetic resonance findings in stress (Takotsubo) cardiomyopathy. JAMA 2011;306:277–86.
13. Templin C, Ghadri JR, Diekmann J, et al. Clinical features and outcomes of Takotsubo (stress) cardiomyopathy. N Engl J Med 2015;373:929–38.
14. Angelini P. Transient left ventricular apical ballooning: a unifying pathophysiologic theory at the edge of Prinzmetal angina. Catheter Cardiovasc Interv 2008;71:342–52.
15. Nojima Y, Kotani J. Global coronary artery spasm caused Takotsubo cardiomyopathy. J Am Coll Cardiol 2010;55:e17.
16. Bybee KA, Prasad A, Barsness GW, et al. Clinical characteristics and thrombolysis in myocardial infarction frame counts in women with transient left ventricular apical ballooning syndrome. Am J Cardiol 2004;94:343–6.
17. Kume T, Akasaka T, Kawamoto T, et al. Assessment of coronary microcirculation in patients with Takotsubo-like left ventricular dysfunction. Circ J 2005;69:934–9.
18. Elesber A, Lerman A, Bybee KA, et al. Myocardial perfusion in apical ballooning syndrome: correlate of myocardial injury. Am Heart J 2006; 152:469.e9-e13.
19. Rigo F, Sicari R, Citro R, et al. Diffuse, marked, reversible impairment in coronary microcirculation in stress cardiomyopathy: a Doppler transthoracic echo study. Ann Med 2009;41:462–70.
20. Galiuto L, De Caterina AR, Porfidia A, et al. Reversible coronary microvascular dysfunction: a common pathogenetic mechanism in apical ballooning or Takotsubo syndrome. Eur Heart J 2010;31:1319–27.

21. Yoshioka T, Hashimoto A, Tsuchihashi K, et al. Clinical implications of midventricular obstruction and intravenous propranolol use in transient left ventricular apical ballooning (Takotsubo cardiomyopathy). Am Heart J 2008;155:526.e1-e7.

22. Mahmoud RE, Mansencal N, Pilliere R, et al. Prevalence and characteristics of left ventricular outflow tract obstruction in Takotsubo syndrome. Am Heart J 2008;156:543-8.

23. Yoshida T, Hibino T, Kako N, et al. A pathophysiologic study of Takotsubo cardiomyopathy with F-18 fluorodeoxyglucose positron emission tomography. Eur Heart J 2007;28:2598-604.

24. Nef HM, Möllmann H, Kostin S, et al. Tako-tsubo cardiomyopathy: intraindividual structural analysis in the acute phase and after functional recovery. Eur Heart J 2007;28:2456-64.

25. Spes C, Knape A, Mudra H. Recurrent Takotsubo like left ventricular dysfunction (apical ballooning) in a patient with pheochromocytoma – a case report. Clin Res Cardiol 2006;95:307-11.

26. Ueda H, Hosokawa Y, Isujii U, et al. An autopsy case of left ventricular apical ballooning probably caused by pheochromocytoma with persistent ST-segment elevation. Int J Cardiol 2011;149:e50-2.

27. Komesaroff PA, Esler MD, Sudhir K. Estrogen supplementation attenuates glucocorticoid and catecholamine responses to mental stress in perimenopausal women. J Clin Endocrinol Metab 1999;84:606-10.

28. Sung BH, Ching M, Izzo JL, et al. Estrogen improves abnormal norepinephrine-induced vasoconstriction in postmenopausal women. J Hypertens 1999;17:523-8.

29. Patel SM, Chokka RG, Prasad K, et al. Distinctive clinical characteristics according to age and gender in apical ballooning syndrome (Takotsubo/stress cardiomyopathy): an analysis focusing on men and young women. J Card Fail 2013;19:306-10.

30. Ueyama T, Hano T, Kasamatsu K, et al. Estrogen attenuates the emotional stress-induced cardiac responses in the animal model of Takotsubo (ampulla) cardiomyopathy. J Cardiovasc Pharmacol 2003;42(Suppl 1):S117-9.

31. Ueyama T, Kasamatsu K, Hano T, et al. Catecholamines and estrogen are involved in the pathogenesis of emotional stress-induced acute heart attack. Ann N Y Acad Sci 2008;1148:479-85.

32. Kuo BT, Choubey R, Novaro GM. Reduced estrogen in menopause may predispose women to Takotsubo cardiomyopathy. Gend Med 2010;7:71-7.

33. Akashi YJ, Nakazawa K, Sakakibara M, et al. ^{123}I-MIBG myocardial scintigraphy in patients with Takotsubo cardiomyopathy. J Nucl Med 2004;45:1121-7.

34. Matsuoka K, Okubo S, Fujii E, et al. Evaluation of the arrhythmogenecity of stress-induced Takotsubo cardiomyopathy from the time course of the 12-lead surface electrocardiogram. Am J Cardiol 2003;92:230-3.

35. Elian D, Osherov A, Matetyky S, et al. Left ventricular apical ballooning: not an uncommon variant of acute myocardial infarction in women. Clin Cardiol 2006;29:9-12.

36. Wedekind H, Möller K, Scholz KH. Takotsubo cardiomyopathy. Incidence in patients with acute coronary syndrome. Herz 2006;31:339-46.

37. Parodi G, Bellandi B, Del Pace S, et al. Natural history of Takotsubo cardiomyopathy. Chest 2011;139:887-92.

38. Deshmukh A, Kumar G, Pant S, et al. Prevalence of Takotsubo cardiomyopathy in the United States. Am Heart J 2012;164:66-71.

39. Lyon AL, Bossone E, Schneider B, et al. Current state of knowledge on Takotsubo syndrome: a position statement from the task force on Takotsubo syndrome of the Heart Failure Association of the European Society of Cardiology. Eur J Heart Fail 2016;18:8-27.

40. Sharkey SW, Windenburg DC, Lesser JR, et al. Natural history and expansive clinical profile of stress (Takotsubo) cardiomyopathy. J Am Coll Cardiol 2010;55:333-41.

41. Brinjikji W, El-Sayed AM, Salka S. In-hospital mortality among patients with Takotsubo cardiomyopathy: a study of the National Inpatient Sample 2008 to 2009. Am Heart J 2012;164:215-21.

42. Song BG, Yang HS, Hwang HK, et al. The impact of stressor patterns on clinical features in patients with Takotsubo cardiomyopathy: experience of two tertiary cardiovascular centers. Clin Cardiol 2012;35:E6-13.

43. Murakami T, Yoshikawa T, Maekawa Y, et al. Gender differences in patients with Takotsubo cardiomyopathy: multi-center registry from Tokyo CCU Network. PLoS One 2015;10(8):e0136655.

44. Kurisu S, Inoue I, Kawagoe T, et al. Presentation of Takotsubo cardiomyopathy in men and women. Clin Cardiol 2010;33:42-5.

45. Schneider B, Athanasiadis A, Stöllberger C, et al. Gender differences in the manifestation of Takotsubo cardiomyopathy. Int J Cardiol 2013;166:584-8.

46. Heer T, Gitt AK, Juenger C, et al. ACOS Investigators. Gender differences in acute non-ST-segment elevation myocardial infarction. Am J Cardiol 2006;98:160-6.

47. Dey S, Flather MD, Devlin G, et al. for the GRACE investigators. Sex related differences in the presentation, treatment and outcomes among patients with acute coronary syndromes: the Global Registry of Acute Coronary Events. Heart 2009;95:20-6.

48. Citro R, Rigo F, Previtali M, et al. Differences in clinical features and in-hospital outcomes of older adults with Takotsubo cardiomyopathy. J Am Geriatr Soc 2012;60:93-8.

49. Schneider B, Athanasiadis A, Schwab J, et al. Complications in the clinical course of Takotsubo cardiomyopathy. Int J Cardiol 2014;176:199–205.

50. Murugiah K, Wang Y, Desai NR, et al. Trends in short- and long-term outcomes for Takotsubo cardiomyopathy among Medicare free-for-service beneficiaries, 2007 to 2012. JACC Heart Fail 2016;4: 197–205.

51. D'Amato N, Colonna P, Brindicci P, et al. Tako-tsubo syndrome in a pregnant woman. Eur J Echocardiogr 2008;9:700–3.

52. Citro R, Giudice R, Mirra M, et al. Is Takotsubo syndrome in the postpartum period a clinical entity different from peripartum cardiomyopathy? J Cardiovasc Med (Hagerstown) 2013;14:568–75.

53. Zdanowicz JA, Utz AC, Bernasconi I, et al. "Broken heart" after cesarean delivery. Case report and review of literature. Arch Gynecol Obstet 2011;283:687–94.

54. Sato A, Yagihara N, Kodama M, et al. Takotsubo cardiomyopathy after delivery in an oestrogen-deficient patient. Int J Cardiol 2011;149:e78–9.

55. Citro R, Giudice R, Mirra M, et al. Takotsubo syndrome soon after caesarean delivery: two case reports. Int J Cardiol 2012;161:e48–9.

56. Haghikia A, Röntgen P, Vogel-Claussen J, et al. Prognostic implication of right ventricular involvement in peripartum cardiomyopathy: a cardiovascular magnetic resonance study. ESC Heart Fail 2015. http://dx.doi.org/10.1002/ehf2.12059.

57. Movahed MR, Mostafizi K. Reverse or inverted left ventricular apical ballooning syndrome (reverse Takotsubo cardiomyopathy) in a young woman in the setting of amphetamine use. Echocardiography 2008;25:429–32.

58. Litvinov IV, Kotowycz MA, Wassmann S. Iatrogenic epinephrine-induced reverse Takotsubo cardiomyopathy: direct evidence supporting the role of catecholamines in the pathophysiology of the "broken heart syndrome". Clin Res Cardiol 2009;98:457–62.

59. Ennezat PV, Pesenti-Rossi D, Aubert JM, et al. Transient left ventricular basal dysfunction without coronary stenosis in acute cerebral disorders: a novel heart syndrome (inverted Takotsubo). Echocardiography 2005;22:599–602.

60. Ramaraj R, Movahed MR. Reverse or inverted Takotsubo cardiomyopathy presents at a younger age compared with the mid or apical variant and is always associated with triggering stress. Congest Heart Fail 2010;16:284–6.

61. Song BG, Chun WJ, Park YH, et al. The clinical characteristics, laboratory parameters, electrocardiographic and echocardiographic findings of reverse or inverted Takotsubo cardiomyopathy: comparison with mid or apical variant. Clin Cardiol 2011;34:693–9.

62. Marti V, Carreras F, Pujadas S, et al. Transient left ventricular basal ballooning – "inverted" Takotsubo. Clin Cardiol 2009;32:E20–1.

63. Ohwada R, Hotta M, Kimura H, et al. Ampulla cardiomyopathy after hypoglycemia in three young female patients with anorexia nervosa. Intern Med 2005;44: 228–33.

64. Hernandez LE. Takotsubo cardiomyopathy: how much do we know of this syndrome in children and young adults? Cardiol Young 2014;24:580–92.

65. Maruyama S, Nomura Y, Fukushige T, et al. Suspected Takotsubo cardiomyopathy caused by withdrawal of bupirenorphine in a child. Circ J 2006; 70:509–11.

66. Olivotti L, Moshiri S, Nicolino A, et al. Stress cardiomyopathy and arrhythmic storm in a 14-year old boy. J Cardiovasc Med (Hagerstown) 2010;11:517–21.

67. Bajolle F, Basquin A, Lucron H, et al. Acute ischemic cardiomyopathy after extreme emotional stress in a child. Congenit Heart Dis 2009;4:387–90.

68. Schoof S, Bertram H, Hohmann D, et al. Takotsubo cardiomyopathy in a 2-year old girl. J Am Coll Cardiol 2010;55:e5.

69. Shaw LJ, Bugiardini R, Merz CN. Women and ischemic heart disease: evolving knowledge. J Am Coll Cardiol 2009;54:1561–75.

70. Patel SM, Lerman A, Lennon R, et al. Impaired coronary microvascular reactivity in women with apical ballooning syndrome (Takotsubo/stress cardiomyopathy). Eur Heart J Acute Cardiovasc Care 2013;2:147–52.

71. Martin EA, Prasad A, Rihal CS, et al. Endothelial function and vascular response to mental stress are impaired in patients with apical ballooning syndrome. J Am Coll Cardiol 2010;56:1840–6.

72. Samuelov-Kinori L, Kinori M, Kogan Y, et al. Takotsubo cardiomyopathy and QT interval prolongation: who are the patients at risk for torsades de pointes? J Electrocardiol 2009;42:353–7.

73. Pilgrim TM, Wyss TR. Takotsubo cardiomyopathy or transient left ventricular apical ballooning syndrome: a systematic review. Int J Cardiol 2008;124:283–92.

74. Dib C, Asirvatham S, Elesber A, et al. Clinical correlates and prognostic significance of electrocardiographic abnormalities in apical ballooning syndrome (Takotsubo/stress-induced cardiomyopathy). Am Heart J 2009;157:933–8.

75. Koeth O, Zahn R, Heer T, et al. Gender differences in patients with acute ST-elevation myocardial infarction complicated by cardiogenic shock. Clin Res Cardiol 2009;98:781–6.

76. Owada M, Aizawa Y, Kurihara K, et al. Risk factors and triggers of sudden death in the working generation: an autopsy proven case-control study. Tohoku J Exp Med 1999;189:245–58.

77. Larsen JA, Kadish AH. Effects of gender on cardiac arrhythmias. J Cardiovasc Electrophysiol 1998;9: 655–64.

78. Singh K, Carson K, Dip LM, et al. Meta-analysis of clinical correlates of acute mortality in Takotsubo cardiomyopathy. Am J Cardiol 2014;113:1420–8.

79. Regnante RA, Zuzek RW, Weinsier SB, et al. Clinical characteristics and four-year outcomes of patients in the Rhode Island Takotsubo Cardiomyopathy Registry. Am J Cardiol 2009;103:1015–9.

80. Chong CR, Neil CJ, Nguyen TH, et al. Dissociation between severity of takotsubo cardiomyopathy and

presentation with shock or hypotension. Clin Cardiol 2013;36:401–6.

81. Schultz T, Shao Y, Redfors B, et al. Stress-induced cardiomyopathy in Sweden: evidence for different ethnic predisposition and altered cardio-circulatory status. Cardiology 2012;122:180–6.

Chronobiology of Takotsubo Syndrome and Myocardial Infarction
Analogies and Differences

Roberto Manfredini, MD[a],*, Fabio Manfredini, MD[b],
Fabio Fabbian, MD[a], Raffaella Salmi, MD[c],
Massimo Gallerani, MD[d],
Eduardo Bossone, MD, PhD, FCCP, FESC, FACC[e],
Abhishek J. Deshmukh, MBBS[f]

KEYWORDS

- Chronobiology, phenomena • Circadian rhythm • Seasons • Day of week • Monday • Gender
- Takotsubo syndrome • Acute myocardial infarction

KEY POINTS

- Takotsubo syndrome (TTS) mimics the clinical scenario of acute myocardial infarction (AMI).
- AMI is characterized by preferred seasonal (winter), day-of-week (Monday), and circadian (morning) peaks of onset.
- Although results are not univocal, TTS seems to exhibit some preferred frequency peaks, with analogies (morning hours and Monday) and differences (summer months).

INTRODUCTION

TTS is a novel acute syndrome characterized by transient left ventricular systolic dysfunction in the absence of significant coronary artery disease, occurring mostly in postmenopausal women after emotional and/or physical stress.[1] TTS is of great interest to cardiologists and emergency medicine physicians, because this condition mimics the clinical scenario of AMI.[2] The reported incidence of TTS based on principal diagnosis at hospital discharge has increased significantly in past years, as shown by data from the Nationwide Inpatient Sample for each of the years from 2006 to 2012. In 2006, 315 cases were recorded, and 6230 cases were recorded in 2012.[3] The increased incidence has been confirmed in a Swedish study of a large sample of subjects confirmed to have TTS in the population of the prospective Swedish Coronary Angiography and Angioplasty Registry (SCAAR), and patients with TTS had short-term and long-term mortality rates similar to those of

This work was supported, in part, by a scientific grant (Fondo Ateneo Ricerca [FAR]) from the University of Ferrara, Italy.

The authors have nothing to disclose.

[a] Clinica Medica Unit, School of Medicine, University of Ferrara, Via Lodovico Ariosto, 35, Ferrara 44121, Italy; [b] Department of Biomedical Sciences and Surgical Specialties, Vascular Diseases Center, School of Medicine, University of Ferrara, Via Lodovico Ariosto, 35, Ferrara 44121, Italy; [c] 2nd Internal Unit of Internal Medicine, General Hospital of Ferrara, Via Aldo Moro 8, Ferrara 44020, Italy; [d] 1st Internal Unit of Internal Medicine, General Hospital of Ferrara, Via Aldo Moro 8, Ferrara 44020, Italy; [e] 'Cava de' Tirreni and Amalfi Coast' Division of Cardiology, Heart Department, University Hospital of Salerno, Via San Leonardo 1, Salerno 84013, Italy; [f] Mayo Clinic Heart Rhythm Section, Cardiovascular Diseases, Mayo Clinic, Rochester, MN 55902, USA

* Corresponding author.

E-mail address: roberto.manfredini@unife.it

Heart Failure Clin 12 (2016) 531–542

http://dx.doi.org/10.1016/j.hfc.2016.06.004

patients with AMI.[4] This observation confirms data from a systematic review and meta-analysis[5] that concluded that TTS is not as benign as once thought, because in-hospital mortality rate among patients with TTS was 4.5%. Older patients with TTS have worse in-hospital outcomes. Data from an Italian cohort of TTS patients showed adverse events (all-cause death, acute heart failure, life-threatening arrhythmias, stroke, and cardiogenic shock) and overall complications were more common in patients aged 75 and older, who showed also a higher in-hospital mortality (6.3%).[6] Out-of-hospital and in-hospital cases of TTS do not seem to be the same entity: (1) patients with in-hospital TTS have more underlying critical diseases and show higher in-hospital mortality than those with out-of-hospital TTS and (2) underlying diseases are significantly associated with higher in-hospital mortality, and cases of in-hospital TTS include a higher proportion of men than those with out-of-hospital TTS.[7] Moreover, men were more likely to have cardiac arrhythmias compared with women (odds ratio [OR] 1.5), and life-threatening cases (ie, ventricular tachycardia and sudden cardiac arrest) were significantly higher in men (ORs 1.7 and 1.6, respectively).[8]

CHRONOBIOLOGIC ASPECTS OF ACUTE MYOCARDIAL INFARCTION AND TAKOTSUBO SYNDROME: ANALOGIES AND DIFFERENCES

Chronobiology is the biomedical science aimed at the study biological rhythms. According to their cycle length, biological rhythms may be divided into 2 main types: (1) ultradian (period <24 hours [eg, hours, minutes, or even seconds]), (2) circadian (period of approximately 24 hours), and (3) infradian (period >24 hours [eg, days, weeks, or months]). Biological rhythms exist at any level of living organisms and persist after million years because they provide an evolutionary advantage, defined *anticipation*, that is, the capacity to know the time of day and arrange metabolic and physiologic resources accordingly. Circadian rhythms are the most commonly and widely studied biological rhythms and are driven by circadian clocks. The principal circadian clock, or master clock, is located in the suprachiasmatic nucleus and is entrained by light.[9] Moreover, other so-called peripheral circadian clocks have been identified. The cardiovascular system is organized in nature according to an oscillatory circadian order, both in conditions of health or disease, and the new concept of chronorisk encompasses the concept that several factors, not harmful if taken alone, are capable of triggering unfavorable events when presenting all together within the same

temporal window.[10] The occurrence of cardiovascular events is not evenly distributed in time but shows peculiar temporal patterns that vary with time of the day, day of the week, and month of the year.[11–13] Both AMI and TTS seem to exhibit some temporal preference in their onset, characterized by variations according to time of the day, day of the week, and month of the year, although with analogies and differences. Each of these temporal frames is discussed, and the available evidence collected by studies of the past 2 decades (1995–2015) is shown in **Tables 1–3**.[14–77]

Circadian

Three decades ago, Muller and colleagues[78] first observed a circadian variation for onset of AMI, characterized by increased morning frequency between 6 AM and 12 AM. Some years later, a meta-analysis considering 30 studies on nonfatal AMI and 19 studies on sudden cardiac death,[79] estimated that nearly 27.7% of morning AMIs and 22.5% of sudden cardiac deaths (approximately 8.8% and 6.8% of all cases, respectively), were attributable to a morning excess of risk. Many studies have given further strong confirmation to this well-known Monday preference (see **Table 1**). Moreover, time of day of onset may also have an impact on on clinical outcome of AMI, because an excess of fatal cases was found between 6 AM and 12 AM, independent of patient age and AMI site or extension.[25]

A series of factors, leading to an increase of oxygen demand and/or reducing oxygen supply, has been shown to be more active during the morning hours. Oxygen demand is increased, for example, by activation of sympathetic nervous system during the rapid eye movement phase of sleep, and by increase of heart rate and blood pressure (BP) on awakening and commencing daily activities. Morning reduction in myocardial oxygen supply may follow the enhanced vascular tone and reduced blood flow and the imbalance between hypercoagulation and reduced endogenous fibrinolysis.[80,81] On one hand, it is likely that AMI and TTS may share some common underlying triggering factors, and, even if characterized by smaller samples of patients, there is also available evidence of a morning preference for TTS (see **Table 1**). Plasma catecholamines, which play a pivotal role in the genesis of TTS, were found significantly higher in a group of patients with TTS compared with patients with AMI.[82] By using a technique assessing muscle sympathetic nerve activity, Vaccaro and colleagues[83] reported for the first time that patients with TTS exhibit elevated sympathetic nervous system activity

Table 1
Circadian onset of acute myocardial infarction & Tako-Tsubo Syndrome (years 1995–2015)

	Author, Year	Country	Cases (n)	Age (y)	Peak
Acute myocardial infarction	Fava et al,[14] 1995	Malta	164	67	No peak
	Fava et al,[14] 1995	Malta	158	66	6–12 AM
	Kono et al,[15] 1996	Japan	608	61 ± 11	7 AM and 8–10 AM
	Krantz et al,[16] 1996	USA	63	62 ± 8	6–11 AM and 2–6 PM
	Spielberg et al,[17] 1996	Germany	1901	68	Retired: 10 AM Working: 10 AM and 4 PM
	Cannon et al,[18] 1997	USA	7730	17%: <65 19%: ≥65	6 AM – noon
	Sayer et al,[19] 1997	UK	1225	62 ± 12	9 AM
	Ku et al,[20] 1998	Taiwan	540	NA	6 AM – noon
	Zhou et al,[21] 1998	China	428	62 ± 11	1–7 AM
	Kinjo et al,[22] 2001	Japan	1,252	50%: <65 50%: ≥65	8 AM – noon
	Yamasaki et al,[23] 2002	Japan	725	67 ± 12	6 AM – noon
	Lopez-Messa et al,[24] 2004	Spain	54,249	10%: <70–40%: ≥70	10 AM
	Manfredini et al,[25] 2004	Italy	442	68 ± 13	8–9 AM
	Tanaka et a,[26] 2004	Japan	174	Rupture group 62 ± 12 Nonrupture group 65 ± 10	6 AM – noon
	Bhalla et al,[27] 2006	India	459	57 ± 5	6 AM – noon and 6 PM – midnight
	Tamura et al,[28] 2006	Japan	21	68 ± 11	6–12 AM
	Mahmoud et al,[29] 2011	USA	124	63 ± 13	7 AM
	Itaya et al,[30] 2012	Japan	522	M 78 ± 18 F 80 ± 16	7–10 AM and 7–9 PM
	Kanth et al,[31] 2013	USA	519	29–94	11:30 AM
	Reavey et al,[32] 2013	Switzerland	361,322	NA	8–9 AM and 5–6 PM
	Wieringa et al,[33] 2014	Netherlands	6970	—	9 AM (onset) midnight – 6 AM (greater infarct size; lower mortality)
	Rallidis et al,[34] 2015	Greece	256	>35	6 AM – noon
	Seneviratna et al,[35] 2015	Singapore	6710	60 ± 13	Midnight – 6 AM
	Fournier et al,[36] 2015	Switzerland	6223	62 ± 12	11 PM (infarct size) midnight (death)
	Mahmoud et al,[37] 2015	Netherlands	6799	NA	3 AM (infarct size)
	Ari et al,[38] 2016	Turkey	252	NA	6 AM – noon
Tako-Tsubo Syndrome	Abdulla et al,[39] 2006	Australia	35	68 ± 13	Morning-afternoon-night (NS)
	Kurisu et al,[40] 2007	Japan	50	72 ± 10	Daytime vs nighttime
	Citro et al,[41] 2009	Italy	88	64 ± 11	Morning
	Mansecal et al,[42] 2010	France	51	71 ± 11	Morning-afternoon
	Sharkey et al,[43] 2012	USA	186	68 ± 14	Midnight – 4 PM
	Song et al,[44] 2013	Korea	137	59 (53 – 72)	Morning

Abbrevistion: NA, not available.

Table 2
Day-of-week onset of acute myocardial infarction & Tako-Tsubo Syndrome (years 1995–2015)

	Author, Year	Country	Cases (n)	Age (y)	Peak
Acute myocardial infarction	van der Palen et al,[45] 1995	Netherland	4983	25–64	Survived: Monday Deceased: Saturday
	Peters et al,[46] 1996	USA	22,516	60	Monday
	Spielberg et al,[17] 1996	Germany	1901	68	Monday
	Sayer et al,[19] 1997	UK	1225	62 ± 12	No peak
	Ku et al,[20] 1998	Taiwan	540	NA	Monday
	Zhou et al,[21] 1998	China	428	62 ± 11	Monday
	Marques-Vidal P et al,[47] 2001	France	17,000	NA	Monday
	Kriszbacher et al,[48] 2008	Hungary	81,215	40%: <65 y 60%: ≥65 y	Monday
	Manfredini et al,[49] 2009	Italy	64,191	M 68 ± 13 F 71 ± 11	Monday
	Reavey et al,[32] 2013	Switzerland	361,322	NA	Monday
	Collart et al,[50] 2014	Belgium	9732	57	Monday
Tako-Tsubo Syndrome	Manfredini et al,[51] 2010	Italy	112	64 ± 11	Monday
	Parodi et al,[52] 2011	Italy	116	73 ± 10	No variation
	Sharkey et al,[43] 2012	USA	186	68 ± 14	Tuesday (NS)
	Song et al,[44] 2013	Korea	137	59 (53–72)	Monday

Abbreviation: NS, not significant.

associated with a decrease in spontaneous baroreflex control of sympathetic activity. A confirmation of the sympathetic neurohormonal hyperreactivity in TTS patients comes also by the demonstration of higher norepinephrine and dopamine levels during mental stress and exercise compared with healthy controls.[84] Catecholamines show a circadian periodicity, with a urinary peak in late morning.[85] Moreover, in healthy women with a routine lifestyle, the excretion of norepinephrine was higher during working hours (9 AM–3 PM).[86] Moreover, catecholamines are stimulated by acute stressful events, and most physical stressors capable of triggering TTS, for example, surgeries, bronchoscopies, endoscopies, and chemotherapy for cancer, are scheduled to take place in the mornings (and least at nights).[44]

Day of Week

Monday represents a critical day for cardiovascular events. Approximately 2 decades ago, Gnecchi-Ruscone and colleagues,[87] in Italy, and Willich and colleagues,[88] in Germany, reported an increased risk of AMI on Monday. A meta-analysis study aimed to quantify the excess risk associated with the Monday peak in cardiovascular mortality found an increased pooled OR of 1.19, without significant differences between subgroups by gender and age.[89] More recently, this Monday preference was confirmed in other studies,[32,48,49] even if the latter was not supported by statistical significance. In addition to AMI, a Monday peak was reported in several series of cases of sudden death,[90,91] in subjects with acute aortic diseases,[92] stroke,[93] and transient ischemic attack.[94]

Selected cardiovascular factors might explain a Monday preference for some cardiovascular events. Morning BP surge, evaluated by means of 24-hour ambulatory monitoring, was the greatest on Monday,[95] and significant differences have been found in blood parameters, characterized by unfavorable profile on Monday compared with non-Monday.[96] Again, the stress of commencing weekly activities has been claimed to play a role. First, Willich and colleagues[88] found the Monday peak was present only in the working but not in nonworking population. A couple of years after, Spielberg and colleagues[17] confirmed the higher frequency of events on Monday but with no differences between working or retired patients. Some years later, a Japanese study confirmed the existence of a main Monday peak in the onset of AMI in working men but found a peak on Saturday for women, hypothesizing the existence of a higher stressful burden for women during weekend.[97] More recently, the weekly peak of AMI was detected on the first workday of the week, with a gradually decreasing tendency until the end of the week. Moreover, there was a significant difference between the number of events on workdays and weekends, but with no

Table 3
Seasonal or monthly onset of acute myocardial infarction & Tako-Tsubo Syndrome (years 1995–2015)

	Author, Year	Country	Cases (n)	Age (y)	Peak
Acute myocardial infarction	Ornato et al,[53] 1996	USA	27,779	NA	Winter–Spring
	Peters et al,[46] 1996	USA	22,516	60.4	Winter
	Spielberg et al,[17] 1996	Germany	2906	68	Winter
	Sayer et al,[19] 1997	UK	1225	62 ± 12	Winter
	Ku et al,[20] 1998	Taiwan	540	NA	No peak
	Spencer et al,[54] 1998	USA	259,891	66	Winter
	Kloner et al,[55] 1999	USA	222,265	NA	Winter
	Sheth et al,[56] 1999	Canada	159,884		Winter
	Grech et al,[57] 2001	Malta	2157	M 62 F 72	Winter
	Yamasaki et al,[23] 2002	Japan	725	67 ± 12	No peak
	Gonzalez Hernandez et al,[58] 2004	Spain	8400	65 ± 12	Winter
	Azegami et al,[59] 2005	Japan	195	20 – 83	Summer
	Manfredini et al,[60] 2005	Italy	4041	M 68 ± 13 F 76±11	Winter
	Morabito et al,[61] 2005	Italy	2683	NA	Winter–Autumn
	Gerber et al,[62] 2006	USA	2676	68 ± 14	No peak
	Rumana et al,[63] 2008	Japan	335	M 68 ± 13 F 75 ± 10	Winter
	Abrignani et al,[64] 2009	Italy	3918	67 ± 8	Winter
	Kriszbacher et al,[65] 2009	Hungary	81,956	NA	Spring
	Manfredini et al,[49] 2009	Italy	64,191	M 68 ± 13 F 71 ± 11	Winter
	Mahmoud et al,[29] 2011	Netherlands	124	63 ± 13	Summer
	Ishikawa et al,[66] 2012	Japan	343	67 ± 13	No peak
	Verberkmoes et al,[67] 2012	Netherlands	11,389	M 64 F 71	Winter
	Reavey et al,[32] 2013	Switzerland	361,322	NA	November–December
	Hong et al,[68] 2014	Korea	265,935		Winter
	Sen et al,[69] 2015	Turkey	402	62 ± 12	Winter
	Lashari et al,[70] 2015	Pakistan	428	49 ± 10	Winter
Tako-Tsubo Syndrome	Hertting et al,[71] 2006	Germany	32	68 (40–85)	Summer (July)
	Abdulla et al,[39] 2006	Australia	35	68 ± 13	Summer (NS)
	Eshterardi et al,[72] 2009	Switzerland	41	65 ± 11	Winter
	Citro et al,[41] 2009	Italy	88	64 ± 11	Summer (July)
	Manfredini et al,[73] 2009	Italy	112	64 ± 11	Summer (July)
	Regnante et al,[74] 2009	USA	70	67 ± 11	Summer
	Mansecal et al,[42] 2010	France	51	71 ± 11	April (p-value NA)
	Summers et al,[75] 2010	USA	186	NA	January & August (NS)
	Parodi et al,[52] 2011	Italy	116	73 ± 10	Spring & Summer (NS)
	Sharkey et al,[43] 2012	USA	186	68 ± 14	December (NS)
	Deshmukh et al,[76] 2012	USA	6837	NA	Summer, July (NS)
	Song et al,[44] 2013	Korea	137	59 (53–72)	Summer (July)
	Aryal et al,[77] 2014	USA	10,989	NA	Late summer–Fall

difference between workers aged less than 65 and pensioners aged greater than 65 or between the 2 genders.[98] In full-time Monday through Saturday working subjects, the molar cortisol-to-dehydroepiandrosterone ratio, measured after awakening, was significantly higher on Monday and Tuesday and significantly lower on Sunday than those on other days.[99] Finally, Collart and colleagues[50] observed that the Monday peak of events was more pronounced in patients ages 35 to 44 and then decreased up to ages of 65 to 69. Thus, other stress factors not necessarily related to work, for example, family roles, could trigger AMI in the younger group.

A limited series of studies is available for TTS and day of week (see **Table 2**). Two studies confirmed a Monday peak,[44–51] 1 found a peak on Tuesday (not statistically significant),[43] and 2 did not find any weekly periodicity.[52]

Seasonal

As for the late 90s, many studies reported the existence of an evident winter preference for onset of AMI (see **Table 3**); data from the US second National Registry of Myocardial Infarction reported 53% more cases in the winter than in the summer, and winter was characterized by the highest frequency of fatal cases.[53] Again, the 30-day mortality of patients hospitalized with AMI in December was higher than in other months, even after specific adjustments.[100]

Potential unfavorable factors could be represented, among others, by (1) seasonal changes in ambient temperature, with consequences on coagulation, BP, and endothelial function; (2) reduction of endothelial function and brachial artery flow-mediated vasodilatation, which is lowest in the winter; and (3) variations in cholesterol levels, with wintertime peaks in plasma levels of total cholesterol and low-density lipoprotein cholesterol.[101] Although a direct effect of cold temperatures on cardiovascular mortality exists,[102] it is possible that this variation may not have an impact on clinical outcome.[103] AMIs that occurred in the United States were found smallest in size during the summer,[104] but European patients with ST-segment elevation myocardial infarction (STEMI) did not show seasonal variations in enzymatic infarct size and 1-year mortality.[105] Several other cardiovascular acute events were shown to exhibit a significant increase in winter, such as aortic aneurysms,[106] stroke,[107] atrial fibrillation,[108] and venous thromboembolism.[109] For some of these cardiovascular diseases, the winter excess of risk has been calculated by means of meta-analysis studies. Venous thromboembolism showed a significantly increased incidence in winter (relative risk [RR] = 1.14),[110] particularly in January (RR = 1.194), and a similar pattern was shown for aortic aneurysm rupture or dissection (December: RR = 1.17; January: RR = 1.14).[111] Several observations reported that such winter preference was independent of patients' underlying comorbid conditions[112] and climate.[113] Convincing evidence, however, supports an opposite seasonal pattern of onset of TTS, characterized by a summer preference (see **Table 3**). No explanations can be given for this phenomenon. However, since catecholamines play an important role in the pathophysiology of TTS, it is interesting that previous studies have reported a summer peak for norepinephrine and epinephrine.[85,86]

DIRECT COMPARATIVE STUDIES

Two studies with direct comparison of patients with AMI and TTS are available. In the Japanese study by Kurisu and colleagues,[40] TTS (n = 37) occurred frequently during 6 AM–noon and 12 PM–6 PM. On the other hand, anterior AMI (n = 544) occurred frequently during 6 AM–12 PM and 6 PM–midnight, and 2 peaks were identified. TTS occurred more frequently in the daytime (6 AM–6 PM) than did anterior AMI (73% vs 49%). More recently, in their single-institution study conducted in the United States on 186 consecutive patients with TTS and 2975 patients with STEMI, Sharkey and colleagues[43] found that TTS events occurred in a circadian pattern with a peak in the afternoon hours, distinctive from the predilection of STEMI for morning hours. The investigators concluded that the different circadian patterns for clinical events identified in TTS compared with STEMI suggest that the 2 conditions may also not share a common pathophysiology. The underlying (but largely undefined) mechanisms responsible for TTS events are most likely linked to environmental triggers in this uniquely susceptible patient population.

ROLE OF STRESS

It is known that TTS occurs mostly in postmenopausal women after emotional and/or physical stress,[1] although recent observation showed that emotional triggers is not as common as physical triggers, and approximately one-third of patients had no evident trigger.[114] In comparison with subjects with acute coronary syndrome, patients who presented with TTS had higher levels of anxiety,[115] and physical stress seems to be more frequent in men, whereas more women experience emotional or no stress.[116] The average score of the Perceived Stress Scale at baseline was found significantly higher for women, explained largely by gender differences in comorbidities, physical and mental health status, intrafamily conflict, caregiving demands, and financial hardship.[117] Common key words for TTS, however, seem to be stress, women, and postmenopause.

Stress, both chronic and acute, is a potential trigger for cardiovascular disease. Acute stressful events (in the recent 48 hours), independent of traditional risk factors, may play a triggering role on the occurrence of acute coronary syndrome, and chronic stress may play a role as well.[118] In an animal model of mice genetically characterized by exacerbated atherosclerosis with spontaneous plaque ruptures, AMI and sudden death, chronic intermittent mental stress (consisting of 3 triggers: water avoidance, damp bedding, and restraint stress) resulted in larger plaques, more coronary stenosis, increased perivascular fibrosis, and higher frequency of AMI.[119] Also in humans, recent findings indicated that long-term stressful circumstances may cause vulnerability to acute psychological or physical stressors and, subsequently, to the onset of TTS.[120]

Living organisms maintain biological homoeostasis during environmental or physiologic challenges and protect from internal or external stress by using mainly 2 mechanisms, the hypothalamic-pituitary-adrenal (HPA) axis, and the sympathetic adrenomedullary system. The HPA axis is activated by corticotropin-releasing hormone (CRH) from the paraventricular nucleus of the hypothalamus, which prompts the release of corticotropin from the pituitary, stimulating the production of glucocorticoids (mainly cortisol) from the adrenal cortex and, to a lesser extent, mineralocorticoids and androgens.[121] The central biological clock controls the HPA axis, creating the diurnal oscillation of circulating adrenocorticotropic hormone and cortisol, and the HPA axis adjusts the circadian rhythmicity of the peripheral clocks in response to various stressors through the glucocorticoid receptor.[122] Cortisol is characterized by the existence of a robust daily rhythm, with circulating cortisol levels exhibiting an early morning peak, then a decline throughout the day, and a nadir at approximately 2 AM–3 AM.[123] Morning cortisol levels may depend, however, on gender and chronotype. After adjusting for basal sex hormones, women have higher morning cortisol.[124] Menopausal transition represents critical moment for women, and insomnia is one of the most disturbing symptoms. In addition to hot flashes, hormones, and psychosocial factors, stress may also play crucial role. In 2 groups of perimenopausal women, with and without insomnia, exposed to experimental presleep stress, women with insomnia exhibited a greater sensitivity to stress, witnessed by increased electroencephalographic arousal and lacked recovery in vagal activity across the stress night.[125] Moreover, cortisol levels are increased after sleep deprivation.[126] Individual differences in chronobiological rhythms may identify a personal chronotype, depending on the diurnal preference, the phase position and period of the circadian rhythms. By means of the Morningness-Eveningness Questionnaire,[127] people may either be morning- or evening-orientated (M-type or E-type) or, in most cases, be neutral chronotype. Chronotypes differ with regards to their sleeping behavior, personality, mental health, and other features. In healthy adults, free cortisol daytime levels were higher in M-type relative to E-type,[128] and, after a stressor-test, E-types had lower salivary cortisol levels and flattened diurnal curve in comparison with M-types.[129] Furthermore, the enhanced physiologic arousal in E-types might contribute to increased vulnerability to psychological distress.[130]

SUMMARY

As for time of onset, AMI and TTS seem to exhibit both analogies (morning and Monday) and differences (winter vs summer). No conclusive data are available to explain such patterns, and gender and age may have influence on chronobiological rhythms. Time of onset does not, however, represent a useful tool in differential diagnosis between TTS and AMI.[131] In a clinical emergency setting, clinical factors (typical chest pain, female gender, postmenopausal age, and possible presence of recent stressful events) as well as instrumental examinations (electrocardiogram, echocardiography, and coronary angiography) play a fundamental role in allowing prompt diagnosis. The identification of temporal frames, however, characterized by highest frequency of onset, could help for a tailored use of drugs,[132] to provide maximal benefit to potentially at risk individuals during the vulnerable periods.

REFERENCES

1. Bossone E, Savarese G, Ferrara F, et al. Takotsubo cardiomyopathy: overview. Heart Failure Clin 2013; 9:249–66.

2. Prasad A, Lerman A, Rihal CS. Apical ballooning syndrome (Tako-Tsubo or stress cardiomyopathy): a mimic of acute myocardial infarction. Am Heart J 2008;155:408–17.

3. Minhas AS, Hughey AB, Kolias TJ. Nationwide trends in reported incidence of Takotsubo Cardiomyopathy from 2006 to 2012. Am J Cardiol 2015; 116:1128–31.

4. Redfors B, Vedad R, Angeras O, et al. Mortality in takotsubo syndrome is similar to mortality in myocardial infarction – A report from the SWEDEHEART registry. Int J Cardiol 2015; 185:282–9.

5. Singh K, Carson K, Shah R, et al. Meta-analysis of clinical correlates of acute mortality in takotsubo cardiomyopathy. Am J Cardiol 2014;113: 1420–8.

6. Citro R, Rigo F, Previtali M, et al. Differences in clinical features and in-hospital outcomes of older adults with tako-tsubo cardiomyopathy. J Am Geriatr Soc 2012;60:93–8.

7. Isogai T, Yasunaga H, Matsui H, et al. Out-of-hospital versus in-hospital Takotsubo cardiomyopathy: analysis of 3719 patients in the Diagnosis Procedure Combination database in Japan. Int J Cardiol 2014;176:413–7.

8. Pant S, Deshmukh A, Mehta K, et al. Burden of arrhythmias in patients with Takotsubo cardiomyopathy (apical ballooning syndrome). Int J Cardiol 2013;170:64–8.

9. Edery I. Circadian rhythms in a nutshell. Physiol Genomics 2000;3:59–74.

10. Portaluppi F, Manfredini R, Fersini C. From a static to a dynamic concept of risk: the circadian epidemiology of cardiovascular events. Chronobiol Int 1999;16:33–49.

11. Fabbian F, Smolensky MH, Tiseo R, et al. Dipper and non-dipper blood pressure 24-hour patterns: circadian rhythm-dependent physiologic and pathophysiologic mechanisms. Chronobiol Int 2013;30: 17–30.

12. Manfredini R, Boari B, Salmi R, et al. Twenty-four-hour patterns in occurrence and pathophysiology of acute cardiovascular events and ischemic heart disease. Chronobiol Int 2013;30:6–16.

13. Smolensky MH, Portaluppi F, Manfredini R, et al. Diurnal and twenty-four hour patterning of human diseases: cardiac, vascular, and respiratory diseases, conditions, and syndromes. Sleep Med Res 2015;21:3–11.

14. Fava S, Azzopardi J, Muscat HA, et al. Absence of circadian variation in the onset of acute myocardial infarction in diabetic subjects. Br Heart J 1995;74: 370–2.

15. Kono T, Morita H, Nishina T, et al. Circadian variations of onset of acute myocardial infarction and efficacy of thrombolytic therapy. J Am Coll Cardiol 1996;27:774–8.

16. Krantz DS, Kop WJ, Gabbay FH, et al. Circadian variation of ambulatory myocardial ischemia. Triggering by daily activities and evidence for an endogenous circadian component. Circulation 1996;93:1364–71.

17. Spielberg C, Falkenhahn D, Willich SN, et al. Circadian, day-of-week, and seasonal variability in myocardial infarction: comparison between working and retired patients. Am Heart J 1996;132:579–85.

18. Cannon CP, McCabe CH, Stone PH, et al. Circadian variation in the onset of unstable angina and non-Q-wave acute myocardial infarction (the TIMI III Registry and TIMI IIIB). Am J Cardiol 1997;79: 253–8.

19. Sayer JW, Wilkinson P, Ranjadayalan K, et al. Attenuation or absence of circadian and seasonal rhythms of acute myocardial infarction. Heart 1997;77:325–9.

20. Ku CS, Yang CY, Lee WJ, et al. Absence of a seasonal variation in myocardial infarction onset in a region without temperature extremes. Cardiology 1998;89:277–82.

21. Zhou RH, Xi B, Gao HQ, et al. Circadian and septadian variation in the occurrence of acute myocardial infarction in a Chinese population. Jpn Circ J 1998;62:190–2.

22. Kinjo K, Sato H, Sato H, et al. Circadian variation of the onset of acute myocardial infarction in the Osaka area, 1998-1999: characterization of morning and nighttime peaks. Jpn Circ J 2001;65: 617–20.

23. Yamasaki F, Seo H, Furuno T, et al. Effect of age on chronological variation of acute myocardial infarction onset: study in Japan. Clin Exp Hypertens 2002;24:1–9.

24. López Messa JB, Garmendia Leiza JR, Aguilar García MD, et al. Cardiovascular risk factors in the circadian rhythm of acute myocardial infarction. Rev Esp Cardiol 2004;57:850–8.

25. Manfredini R, Boari B, Bressan S, et al. Influence of circadian rhythm on mortality after myocardial infarction: data from a prospective cohort of emergency calls. Am J Emerg Med 2004;22:555–9.

26. Tanaka A, Kawarabayashi T, Fukuda D, et al. Circadian variation of plaque rupture in acute myocardial infarction. Am J Cardiol 2004;93:1–5.

27. Bhalla A, Sachdev A, Lehl SS, et al. Ageing and circadian variation in cardiovascular events. Singapore Med J 2006;47:305–8.

28. Tamura A, Watanabe T, Nagase K, et al. Circadian variation in symptomatic subacute stent thrombosis after bare metal coronary stent implantation. Am J Cardiol 2006;97:195–7.

29. Mahmoud KD, Lennon RJ, Ting HH, et al. Circadian variation in coronary stent thrombosis. JACC Cardiovasc Interv 2011;4:183–90.

30. Itaya H, Takagi T, Sugi K, et al. Contents of second peak in the circadian variation of acute myocardial infarction in the Japanese population. J Cardiol 2012;59:147–53.

31. Kanth R, Ittaman S, Rezkalla S. Circadian patterns of ST elevation myocardial infarction in the new millennium. Clin Med Res 2013;11:66–72.

32. Reavey M, Saner H, Paccaud F, et al. Exploring the periodicity of cardiovascular events in Switzerland: variation in deaths and hospitalizations across seasons, day of the week and hour of the day. Int J Cardiol 2013;168:2195–200.

33. Wieringa WG, Lexis CP, Mahmoud KD, et al. Time of symptom onset and value of myocardial blush and infarct size on prognosis in patients with ST-elevation myocardial infarction. Chronobiol Int 2014;31:797–806.

34. Rallidis LS, Triantafyllis AS, Sakadakis EA, et al. Circadian pattern of symptoms onset in patients ≤35 years presenting with ST-segment elevation acute myocardial infarction. Eur J Intern Med 2015;26:607–10.

35. Seneviratna A, Lim GH, Devi A, et al. Circadian dependence of infarct size and acute heart failure in ST elevation myocardial infarction. PLoS One 2015;10:e0128526.

36. Fournier S, Taffé P, Radovanovic D, et al. Myocardial infarct size and mortality depend on the time of day-a large multicenter study. PLoS One 2015; 10:e0119157.

37. Mahmoud KD, Nijsten MW, Wieringa WG, et al. Independent association between symptom onset time and infarct size in patients with ST-elevation myocardial infarction undergoing primary percutaneous coronary intervention. Chronobiol Int 2015; 32:468–77.

38. Arı H, Sonmez O, Koc F, et al. Circadian rhythm of infarct size and left ventricular function evaluated with tissue doppler echocardiography in ST elevation myocardial infarction. Heart Lung Circ 2016; 25:250–6.

39. Abdulla I, Kay S, Mussap C, et al. Apical sparing in tako-tsubo cardiomyopathy. Intern Med J 2006;36: 414–8.

40. Kurisu S, Inoue I, Kawagoe T, et al. Circadian variation in the occurrence of tako-tsubo cardiomyopathy: comparison with acute myocardial infarction. Int J Cardiol 2007;115:270–1.

41. Citro R, Previtali M, Bovelli D, et al. Chronobiological patterns of onset of Tako-Tsubo cardiomyopathy: a multicenter Italian study. J Am Coll Cardiol 2009;54:180–1.

42. Mansencal N, El Mahmoud R, Dubourg O. Occurrence of Tako-Tsubo cardiomyopathy and chronobiological variation. J Am Coll Cardiol 2010;55: 500–1 [author reply: 501–2].

43. Sharkey SW, Lesser JR, Garberich RF, et al. Comparison of circadian rhythm patterns in Takotsubo cardiomyopathy versus ST-segment elevation myocardial infarction. Am J Cardiol 2012;110: 795–9.

44. Song BG, Oh JH, Kim HJ, et al. Chronobiological variation in the occurrence of Tako-tsubo cardiomyopathy: experiences of two tertiary cardiovascular centers. Heart Lung 2013;42:40–7.

45. van der Palen J, Doggen CJ, Beaglehole R. Variation in the time and day of onset of myocardial infarction and sudden death. N Z Med J 1995;108:332–4.

46. Peters RW, Brooks MM, Zoble RG, et al. Chronobiology of acute myocardial infarction: cardiac arrhythmia suppression trial (CAST) experience. Am J Cardiol 1996;78:1198–201.

47. Marques-Vidal P, Arveiler D, Amouyel P, et al. Myocardial infarction rates are higher on weekends than on weekdays in middle aged French men. Heart 2001;86:341–2.

48. Kriszbacher I, Boncz I, Koppán M, et al. Seasonal variations in the occurrence of acute myocardial infarction in Hungary between 2000 and 2004. Int J Cardiol 2008;129:251–4.

49. Manfredini R, Manfredini F, Boari B, et al. Seasonal and weekly patterns of hospital admissions for nonfatal and fatal myocardial infarction. Am J Emerg Med 2009;27:1097–103.

50. Collart P, Coppieters Y, Godin I, et al. Day-of-the-week variations in myocardial infarction onset over a 27-year period: the importance of age and other risk factors. Am J Emerg Med 2014;32:558–62.

51. Manfredini R, Citro R, Previtali M, et al. Monday preference in onset of takotsubo cardiomyopathy. Am J Emerg Med 2010;28:715–9.

52. Parodi G, Bellandi B, Del Pace S, et al. Natural history of tako-tsubo cardiomyopathy. Chest 2011; 139:887–92.

53. Ornato JP, Peberdy MA, Chandra NC, et al. Seasonal pattern of acute myocardial infarction in the National Registry of Myocardial Infarction. J Am Coll Cardiol 1996;28:1684–8.

54. Spencer FA, Goldberg RJ, Becker RC, et al. Seasonal distribution of acute myocardial infarction in the second National Registry of Myocardial Infarction. J Am Coll Cardiol 1998;31:1226–33.

55. Kloner RA, Poole WK, Perritt RL. When throughout the year is coronary death most likely to occur? A 12-year population-based analysis of more than 220 000 cases. Circulation 1999;100:1630–4.

56. Sheth T, Nair C, Muller J, et al. Increased winter mortality from acute myocardial infarction and stroke: the effect of age. J Am Coll Cardiol 1999; 33:1916–9.

57. Grech V, Aquilina O, Pace J. Gender differences in seasonality of acute myocardial infarction admissions and mortality in a population-based study. J Epidemiol Community Health 2001;55:147–8.

58. González Hernández E, Cabadés O'Callaghan A, Cebrián Doménech J, et al. Seasonal variations in admissions for acute myocardial infarction. The PRIMVAC study. Rev Esp Cardiol 2004;57: 12–9.

59. Azegami M, Hongo M, Yazaki Y, et al. Seasonal difference in onset of coronary heart disease in young Japanese patients: a comparison with older patients. Circ J 2005;69:1176–9.

60. Manfredini R, Boari B, Smolensky MH, et al. Seasonal variation in onset of myocardial infarction-a 7-year single-center study in Italy. Chronobiol Int 2005;22:1121–35.

61. Morabito M, Modesti PA, Cecchi L, et al. Relationships between weather and myocardial infarction: a biometeorological approach. Int J Cardiol 2005; 105:288–93.

62. Gerber Y, Jacobsen SJ, Killian JM, et al. Seasonality and daily weather conditions in relation to myocardial infarction and sudden cardiac death in Olmsted County, Minnesota, 1979 to 2002. J Am Coll Cardiol 2006;48:287–92.

63. Rumana N, Kita Y, Turin TC, et al. Seasonal pattern of incidence and case fatality of acute myocardial infarction in a Japanese population (from the Takashima AMI Registry, 1988 to 2003). Am J Cardiol 2008;102:1307–11.

64. Abrignani MG, Corrao S, Biondo GB, et al. Influence of climatic variables on acute myocardial infarction hospital admissions. Int J Cardiol 2009; 137:123–9.

65. Kriszbacher I, Bódis J, Csoboth I, et al. The occurrence of acute myocardial infarction in relation to weather conditions. Int J Cardiol 2009;135:136–8.

66. Ishikawa K, Niwa M, Tanaka T. Difference of intensity and disparity in impact of climate on several vascular diseases. Heart Vessels 2012;27:1–9.

67. Verberkmoes NJ, Soliman Hamad MA, Ter Woorst JF, et al. Impact of temperature and atmospheric pressure on the incidence of major acute cardiovascular events. Neth Heart J 2012;20: 193–6.

68. Hong JS, Kang HC. Seasonal variation in case fatality rate in Korean patients with acute myocardial infarction using the 1997-2006 Korean National Health Insurance Claims Database. Acta Cardiol 2014;69:513–21.

69. Sen T, Astarcioglu MA, Asarcikli LD, et al. The effects of air pollution and weather conditions on the incidence of acute myocardial infarction. Am J Emerg Med 2016;34(3):449–54.

70. Lashari MN, Alam MT, Khan MS, et al. Variation in admission rates of acute coronary syndrome patients in coronary care unit according to different seasons. J Coll Physicians Surg Pak 2015;25:91–4.

71. Hertting K, Krause K, Härle T, et al. Transient left ventricular apical ballooning in a community hospital in Germany. Int J Cardiol 2006;112:282–8.

72. Eshtehardi P, Koestner SC, Adorjan P, et al. Transient apical ballooning syndrome–clinical characteristics, ballooning pattern, and long-term follow-up in a Swiss population. Int J Cardiol 2009;135:370–5.

73. Manfredini R, Citro R, Previtali M, et al. Summer preference in the occurrence of takotsubo cardiomyopathy is independent of age. J Am Geriatr Soc 2009;57:1509–11.

74. Regnante RA, Zuzek RW, Weinsier SB, et al. Clinical characteristics and four-year outcomes of patients in the Rhode Island Takotsubo Cardiomyopathy Registry. Am J Cardiol 2009;103:1015–9.

75. Summers MR, Dib C, Prasad A. Chronobiology of Tako-tsubo cardiomyopathy (apical ballooning syndrome). J Am Geriatr Soc 2010;58:805–6.

76. Deshmukh A, Kumar G, Pant S, et al. Prevalence of Takotsubo cardiomyopathy in the United States. Am Heart J 2012;164:66–71.e1.

77. Aryal MR, Pathak R, Karmacharya P, et al. Seasonal and regional variation in Takotsubo cardiomyopathy. Am J Cardiol 2014;113:1592.

78. Muller JE, Stone PH, Turi ZG, et al. Circadian variation in the frequency of onset of acute myocardial infarction. N Engl J Med 1985;313:1315–22.

79. Cohen MC, Rohtla KM, Lavery CE, et al. Meta-analysis of the morning excess of acute myocardial infarction and sudden cardiac death. Am J Cardiol 1997;79:1512–5.

80. Manfredini R, Gallerani M, Portaluppi F, et al. Relationships of the circadian rhythms of thrombotic, ischemic, hemorrhagic, and arrhythmic events to blood pressure rhythms. Ann N Y Acad Sci 1996; 783:141–58.

81. Manfredini R, Boari B, Salmi R, et al. Circadian variation of cardiovascular events and morning blood pressure surge. Vasc Dis Prev 2008;5:246 51.

82. Wittstein IS, Thiemann DR, Lima JAC, et al. Neurohumoral features of myocardial stunning due to sudden emotional stress. N Engl J Med 2005;352: 539–48.

83. Vaccaro A, Despas F, Delmas C, et al. Direct evidences for sympathetic and baroreflex impairment in Tako Tsubo cardiomyopathy. PLos One 2014;9:e93278.

84. Smeijers L, Szabò BM, van Dammen L, et al. Emotional, neurohormonal, and hemodynamic responses to mental stress in Tako-Tsubo cardiomyopathy. Am J Cardiol 2015;115:1580–6.

85. Descovich GC, Montalbetti N, Kiahl JF, et al. Age and catecholamine rhythms. Chronobiologia 1974;1:163–71.

86. Hansen AM, Garde AH, Skovgaard LT, et al. Seasonal and biological variation of urinary epinephrine, norepinephrine, and cortisol in healthy women. Clin Chim Acta 2001;309:25–35.

87. Gnecchi-Ruscone T, Piccaluga E, Guzzetti S, et al. Morning and Monday:critical periods for the onset of acute myocardial infarction. Eur Heart J 1994; 15:882–7.

88. Willich SN, Lowel H, Lewis M, et al. Weekly variation of acute myocardial infarction. Increased Monday risk in the working population. Circulation 1994;90:87–93.

89. Witte DR, Grobbee DR, Bots ML, et al. A meta-analysis of excess cardiac mortality on Monday. Eur J Epidemiol 2005;20:401–6.

90. Arntz HR, Willich SN, Schreiber C, et al. Diurnal, weekly, and seasonal variation of sudden death. Population-based analysis of 24,061 consecutive cases. Eur Heart J 2000;21:315–20.

91. Gruska M, Gaul GB, Winkler M, et al. Increased occurrence of out-of-hospital cardiac arrest on

Mondays in a community-based study. Chronobiol Int 2005;20:401–6.

92. Manfredini R, Boari B, Salmi R, et al. Day-of-week variability in the occurrence and outcome of aortic diseases: does it exist? Am J Emerg Med 2008;26: 363–6.

93. Manfredini R, Casetta I, Paolino E, et al. Monday preference in onset of ischemic stroke. Am J Med 2001;111:401–3.

94. Manfredini R, Manfredini F, Boari B, et al. Temporal patterns of hospital admissions for transient ischemic attack: a retrospective population-based study in the Emilia-Romagna region of Italy. Clin Appl Thromb Hemost 2010;16:153–60.

95. Murakami S, Otsuka K, Kubo Y, et al. Repeated ambulatory monitoring reveals a Monday morning surge in blood pressure in a community-dwelling population. Am J Hypertens 2004;17: 1179–83.

96. Urdal P, Anderssen SA, Holme I, et al. Monday and non-Monday concentrations of lifestyle-related blood components in the Oslo Diet and Exercise Study. J Intern Med 1998;244:507–13.

97. Kinjo K, Sato H, Sato H, et al. Variation during the week in the incidence of acute myocardial infarction: increased risk for Japanese women on Saturdays. Heart 2003;89:398–403.

98. Bodis J, Boncz I, Kriszbacher I. Permanent stress may be trigger of an acute myocardial infarction on the first work-day of the week. Int J Cardiol 2010;144:423–5.

99. Kim MS, Lee YJ, Ahn RS. Day-to-day differences in cortisol levels and molar cortisol-to-DHEA ratios among working individuals. Yonsei Med J 2010; 51:212–8.

100. Meine TJ, Patel MR, DePuy V, et al. Evidence-based therapies and mortality in patients hospitalized in December with acute myocardial infarction. Ann Intern Med 2005;143:481–5.

101. Manfredini R, Manfredini F, Malagoni AM, et al. Chronobiology of vascular disorders: a "seasonal" link between arterial and venous thrombotic diseases? J Coagul Disord 2010;2:61–7.

102. Wilmhurst P. Temperature and cardiovascular mortality. BMJ 1994;309:1029–30.

103. Mehta RH, Manfredini R, Bossone E, et al. Does circadian and seasonal variation occurrence of acute aortic dissection influence in-hospital mortality? Chronobiol Int 2005;22:343–51.

104. Kloner RA, Das S, Poole K, et al. Seasonal variation of myocardial infarction size. Am J Cardiol 2001;88: 1021–4.

105. De Luca G, Suryapranata H, Ottervanger JP, et al. Absence of seasonal variation in myocardial infarction, enzymatic infarct size, and mortality in patients with ST-segment elevation treated with primary angioplasty. Am J Cardiol 2005;95:1459–61.

106. Mehta RH, Manfredini R, Hassan F, et al. Chronobiologic patterns of acute aortic dissection. Circulation 2002;106:1110–5.

107. Manfredini R, Gallerani M, Portaluppi F, et al. Chronobiological patterns of onset of acute cerebrovascular diseases. Thromb Res 1997;88:451–63.

108. Deshmukh AJ, Pant S, Kumar G, et al. Seasonal variations in atrial fibrillation related hospitalizations. Int J Cardiol 2013;168:1555–6.

109. Gallerani M, Boari B, Smolensky MH, et al. Seasonal variation in occurrence of pulmonary embolism: analysis of the database of the Emilia-Romagna region. Italy Chronobiol Int 2007;24: 143–60.

110. Dentali F, Ageno W, Rancan E, et al. Seasonal and monthly variability in the incidence of venous thromboembolism. A systematic review and a meta-analysis of the literature. Thromb Haemost 2011;106:439–47.

111. Vitale J, Manfredini R, Gallerani M, et al. Chronobiology of acute aortic rupture or dissection: a systematic review and a meta-analysis of the literature. Chronobiol Int 2015;32:385–94.

112. Manfredini R, Gallerani M, Boari B, et al. Seasonal variation in onset of pulmonary embolism is independent of patients' underlying risk comorbid conditions. Clin Appl Thromb Hemost 2004;10: 39–43.

113. Mehta RH, Manfredini R, Bossone E, et al. The winter peak in the occurrence of acute aortic dissection is independent of climate. Chronobiol Int 2005;22:723–9.

114. Templin C, Ghadri JR, Diekmann J, et al. Clinical features and outcomes of Takotsubo (Stress) Cardiomyopathy. N Engl J Med 2015;373:929–38.

115. Goh AC, Wong S, Zaroff JG, et al. Comparing anxiety and depression in patients with Takotsubo stress cardiomyopathy to those with acute coronary syndrome. J Cardiopulm Rehabil Prev 2016; 36:106–11.

116. Schneider B, Athanasiadis A, Stollberger C, et al. Gender differences in the manifestation of takotsubo cardiomyopathy. Int J Cardiol 2013;166: 584–8.

117. Xu X, Bao H, Strait K, et al. Sex differences in perceived stress and early recovery in young and middle-aged patients with acute myocardial infarction. Circulation 2015;131:614–23.

118. Roohafza H, Talaei M, Sadeghi M, et al. Association between acute and chronic life events on acute coronary syndrome: a case-control study. J Cardiovasc Nurs 2010;25:E1–7.

119. Roth L, Rombouts M, Schrijvers DM, et al. Chronic intermittent mental stress promotes atherosclerotic plaque vulnerability, myocardial infarction and sudden death in mice. Atherosclerosis 2015;242:288–94.

120. Wallstrom S, Ulin K, Maatta S, et al. Impact of long-term stress in Takotsubo syndrome: experience of patients. Eur J Cardiovasc Nurs 2015 [pii:1474515115618568; Epub ahead of print].

121. Mathe G. The need of a physiologic and pathophysiologic definition of stress. J Psychosom Res 2000;54:119–21.

122. Kino T. Circadian rhythms of glucocorticoid hormone actions in target tissues: potential clinical implications. Sci Signal 2012;5:pt4.

123. Van Cauter E, Leproult R, Kupfer DJ. Effects of gender and age on the levels and circadian rhythmicity of plasma cortisol. J Clin Endocrinol Metab 1996;8:2468–73.

124. Juster RP, Raymond C, Desrchers AB, et al. Sex hormones adjust 'sex-specific' reactive and diurnal cortisol profiles. Psychoneuroendocrinology 2016; 63:282–90.

125. Zambotti M, Sugarbaker D, Trinder J, et al. Acute stress alters autonomic modulation during sleep in women approaching menopause. Psychoneuroendocrinology 2015;66:1–10.

126. Wright KP Jr, Drake AL, Frey DJ, et al. Influence of sleep deprivation and circadian misalignment on cortisol, inflammatory markers, and cytokine balance. Brain Behav Immun 2015;47:24–34.

127. Horne JA, Ostberg O. A self-assessment questionnaire to determine morningness-eveningness in human circadian rhythms. Int J Chronobiol 1976; 4:97–110.

128. Kudielka BM, Bellingrath S, Hellhammer DH. Further support for higher salivary cortisol levels in 'morning' compared to 'evening' persons. J Psychosom Res 2007;62:595–6.

129. Oginska H, Fafrowicz M, Golonka K, et al. Chronotype, sleep loss, and diurnal pattern of salivary cortisol in a simulated daylong driving. Chronobiol Int 2010;27:959–74.

130. Roeser K, Obergfell F, Meule A, et al. Of larks and hearts–morningness/eveningness, heart rate variability, and cardiovascular stress response at different times of day. Physiol Behav 2012;106: 151–7.

131. Manfredini R, Eagle KA, Bossone E. Acute myocardial infarction and Tako-tsubo cardiomyopathy: could time of onset help to diagnose? Exp Rev Cardiovasc Ther 2011;9:123–6.

132. De Giorgi A, Mallozzi Menegatti A, Fabbian F, et al. Circadian rhythm and medical diseases: does it matter when drugs are taken? Eur J Intern Med 2013;24:698–706.

Takotsubo Syndrome and Embolic Events

Ibrahim El-Battrawy, MD[a,b], Martin Borggrefe, MD[a,b], Ibrahim Akin, MD[a,b],*

KEYWORDS

- Takotsubo cardiomyopathy • Thromboembolic events • Ventricular thrombus • Stroke

KEY POINTS

- Thromboembolism is a common complication of takotsubo cardiomyopathy (TTC).
- Patients present initially with symptoms such as chest pain and dyspnea.
- Close follow-up of patients with TTC is important to avoid overlooking this serious complication.
- There is a need for individualized therapy.

INTRODUCTION

Takotsubo cardiomyopathy (TTC), a well-known reversible disease predominantly affecting post-menopausal women,[1] was first described in 1990. It is usually precipitated by a transient apical ballooning of the left ventricle (LV) with wall motion abnormalities of the middistal and apical regions and is associated with a decreased ejection fraction. Additionally, the involvement of the right ventricle (RV) has also been described in up to 18.6% of patients.[2,3] The spontaneous recovery of stunned myocardial muscle in TTC, however, is generally observed within days or weeks.

Patients present initially with symptoms such as chest pain and dyspnea. This could mimic an acute coronary syndrome (ACS) and admitted patients are commonly treated as having suffered from one. TTC has also been associated with some critical complications such as heart failure, life-threatening arrhythmias, atrial fibrillation, prolonged QT interval, thromboembolic events, recurrence of TTC, LV outflow obstruction, mitral valve regurgitation, and cardiac rupture.[4–9] Interestingly, the in-hospital mortality rate of TTC is similar to that of ACS.[10]

We sought to determine the epidemiologic as well as the clinical aspects of thromboembolic events in TTC.[4,11–16]

INCIDENCE OF THROMBOEMBOLIC EVENTS IN TAKOTSUBO CARDIOMYOPATHY

The incidence and clinical significance of thromboembolic events in TTC has not yet been established sufficiently. Data documenting these events are scarce and recent literature highlights only a few isolated case reports.[4,11–26]

An in-depth analysis of existing references, however, does reveal the common occurrence of intraventricular thrombus (**Fig. 1**), signifying potential relevance in many of the thromboembolic events. For example, cerebral ischemic stroke (**Fig. 2**), following to the development of a thrombus in a patient with TTC, has been reported recently in the literature. In rare cases, thromboembolic events may present as emboli in the peripheral arterial system, such as the radial, renal, pulmonary, and popliteal arteries. The incidence of ventricular thrombus formation and stroke varies between 2.5% and 8% and 1% and 5%, respectively.[4,10,14,16]

Conflict of Interest: None.

[a] First Department of Medicine, Medical Faculty Mannheim, University Heidelberg, Theodor-Kutzer-Ufer 1-3, Mannheim 68167, Germany; [b] DZHK (German Center for Cardiovascular Research), Partner Site, Heidelberg-Mannheim, Theodor-Kutzer-Ufer 1-3, Mannheim 68167, Germany
* Corresponding author. First Department of Medicine, University Medical Centre Mannheim, Theodor-Kutzer-Ufer 1-3, Mannheim 68167, Germany.
E-mail address: Ibrahim.Akin@UMM.de

Heart Failure Clin 12 (2016) 543–550
http://dx.doi.org/10.1016/j.hfc.2016.06.011
1551-7136/16/$ – see front matter © 2016 Elsevier Inc. All rights reserved.

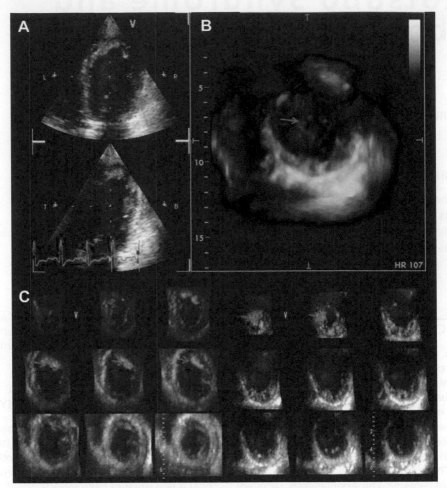

Fig. 1. (*A*, *B*) Echocardiography of patients with apical takotsubo cardiomyopathy showing a left ventricular thrombus formation. (*C*) A 4-dimensional full-volume dataset was used to slice the left ventricle into 9 equidistant short-axis views.

PATHOPHYSIOLOGY OF TAKOTSUBO CARDIOMYOPATHY AND RELATED EMBOLIC EVENTS

TTC occurs predominantly in postmenopausal women and the disease is usually provoked by emotional or physical stress.[1–3,27] An enhanced sympathetic activity with an elevation of catecholamine levels has been documented in these patients.[28] Furthermore, coronary vasospasm and widespread coronary microvascular dysfunction might be a contributing factor to the pathophysiologic mechanism of TTC.[29,30] Nevertheless, a defining explanation to its underlying pathogenesis remains unresolved. In general, ventricular thrombus can occur in the setting of ventricular dysfunction, especially in the acute stage after myocardial infarction,[31,32] noncompaction cardiomyopathy, dilated cardiomyopathy,[33,34] antiphospholipid antibody syndrome, hypereosinophilic syndrome, and autoimmune disorders

like Adamantiadis-Behcet's disease and lupus erythematosus.[35–38] In TTC, the development of an acute ventricular thrombus is presumably explained by the triad of Virchow, outlining as cause in this scenario the low blood flow in the ventricle. The improvement of wall motion abnormality in TTC might promote discharge of this intraventricular thrombus into the peripheral bloodstream, thus initiating an embolic event.[24] Another hypothesis involving the coagulation cascade has also been proposed recently as the underlying mechanism contributing to the development of thromboemboli in patients with TTC.[39] Several endothelial markers and clotting activation biomarkers (von Willebrand factor and plasminogen) as well as lipoprotein A levels were higher in patients with TTC compared with the healthy population suggesting a role of endothelial dysfunction and similar pathologies contributing to the hyperviscosity of blood flow in TTC.[40]

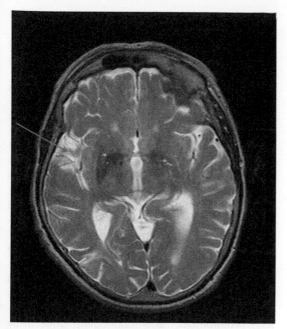

Fig. 2. MR tomogram shows watershed cerebral infarction (*arrow*) in a patient with takotsubo cardiomyopathy.

DIAGNOSTIC CHALLENGE

There are many inherent difficulties in confirming intraventricular thrombus formation and its peripheral embolization in TTC. Although 2-dimensional echocardiography and transesophageal echocardiography remains the gold standard, the number of echocardiograms performed per patient, time point, operator skills, and use of contrast agents may all influence the sensitivity and specificity of this tool in thrombus detection. The majority of thrombi occur in the LV apex; however, other sites may also be affected. For this reason, the area adjacent to the papillary muscles, which seems especially prone to develop thrombus, should be examined carefully.[4,14] In rare cases, RV involvement with concomitant thrombus formation might also be seen.[41] An inherent diagnostic hurdle is the difficulty in differentiating thrombus formation from a tumor, as well as the possibility of overlooking smaller thrombi in echocardiography.[17,42,43] Some study groups have suggested the use of computed tomography and cardiac MRI to rule out intraventricular thrombus.[17,43] Patients presenting with symptoms of a stroke, with a supposed cardiac emboli as source of origin, have been recommended cardiac MRI in addition to a cranial computed tomography.[21,25] In the case of a mechanically ventilated patient, embolization could also be easily overlooked owing to the masked nature of its presenting signs and symptoms. A high degree of clinical skill and interpretation would be a prerequisite in this scenario.

THERAPEUTIC APPROACH

A review of the current literature reveals that most patients with TTC suffering from thrombus formation have been treated with anticoagulants like warfarin and/or heparin. However, the type of anticoagulant drug prescribed was variable and details as to the dosage and therapy duration was often not reported.

Patients suffering from cerebral ischemia or stroke were treated with thrombolysis or platelet inhibitors according to the time of symptom onset.[21,25,44] In very rare cases, surgical treatment was recommended for patients with unstable LV thrombus and for those with presence of thrombus despite therapeutic anticoagulation.[45,46] Patients developing peripheral embolization were treated with balloon angioplasty, platelet inhibitors, and anticoagulation drugs such as warfarin and/or heparin. In the rare event of patients developing limb ischemia, a surgical thrombectomy or a percutaneous transluminal angioplasty was performed and in certain cases amputation of the extremity was also necessary.[47] This highlights the need for an individualized therapeutic approach, which is discussed and ascertained by an interdisciplinary team composed of a cardiologist, neurologist, and surgeons.

FOLLOW-UP AND MANAGEMENT OF PATIENTS WITH THROMBUS FORMATION IN LIGHT OF TAKOTSUBO CARDIOMYOPATHY

In the event of ventricular thrombus formation in a TTC patient, it is likely that this was present at the time of diagnosis. However, recent case reports have suggested the development of LV thrombus much later in the course of the disease.[4,11,13,48,49] This pattern of presentation underscores the need for close follow-up with echocardiography and cardiac MRI. In special scenarios, even a computed tomography scan could provide valuable insight and detail. Patients should be informed about their diagnosis and the need for urgent management has to be explained succinctly.

The inherent risk of thrombus formation and the initiation of the embolic event is not mitigated completely with anticoagulant therapy. These events could still develop in the course of the disease process. In such cases, it is pertinent to rule out a hematologic disease or neoplasia with necessary diagnostic tests and the management of these patients would be based on an individualized concept.

DISCUSSION

TTC, initially described in Japanese populations, occurs predominantly in postmenopausal women and the disease is usually provoked by emotional or physical stress. Enhanced sympathetic activity with elevation of catecholamine levels has been documented in these patients[1] Furthermore, coronary vasospasm and widespread coronary microvascular dysfunction might be a contributing factor in the pathophysiologic mechanism of TTC. Nevertheless, a defining explanation to its' underlying pathogenesis remains unresolved.

Although TTC is now encountered as a benign disease, the in-hospital mortality is as high as 1% to 4%. Moreover, other TTC-related complications such as congestive heart failure, cardiogenic shock, respiratory distress, and lethal arrhythmias have also been reported.[4–9]

Because of a lack of sufficient data in the published literature, it is difficult to draw definitive conclusions to a TTC syndrome encompassing the formation of a ventricular thrombus, development of a stroke, or peripheral embolization.[2,16,20,30,50–54]

The incidence of LV thrombus formation is at least 5% in patients with ischemic heart disease. This value corresponds with those diagnosed with TTC and could also possibly be an underestimate.[2,4,55–57] These findings confirm that the occurrence of ventricular thrombus formation is not significantly different in these 2 unique categories of patients. It has been noted that patients diagnosed with an acute myocardial infarction or with TTC, and who develop LV thrombosis, have increased levels of C-reactive protein. This could explain a potential pathogenic role of inflammation in the process of thrombus formation.[4,58] It is possible that, in the acute phase, there is no difference in the development of thrombosis between ACS and patients with TTC, because there is a similar impairment and stasis of blood flow in the ventricle with a stunned myocardium. However, the rate of embolization might be higher in patients with TTC because the recovery from impaired LV function is much earlier than in the setting of an acute myocardial infarction. In the long term, the risk of thromboembolism might be reversed, with higher incidence rates in patients with an acute myocardial infarction and this can be attributed to the sustained hypokinesia or akinesia of the myocardium.

Echocardiography is the gold standard in the diagnosis of ventricular thrombus formation. The use of contrast agents is suggested in uncertain cases. It is widely known that the RV is involved in as many as 18.5% of all TTC cases.[2,3] However, there is little literature documenting thrombus formation in the RV in patients suffering from TTC.

Cerebral embolism might result from LV thrombosis in TTC. However, there have also been reports indicating stroke in patients in the absence of ventricular thrombus.[59] A possible explanation is that TTC might be the consequence of stroke-related stress. Cerebral ischemia in itself may be the cause of a neurocardiac injury syndrome as seen in some patients with subarachnoid hemorrhage.[60] This stress-related phenomenon has been reported in patients after surgery.

The documentation of the clinical course is an important factor for etiologic purposes.[16,21] It has been reported that patients with TTC present with cerebral events at an annual rate of up to 1.7%. These data necessitate a close follow-up of all patients with TTC.[10] An interesting contrast is the data from previous randomized controlled trials, which revealed that 4.6% of patients with ACS had experienced a stroke on follow-up.[61]

A hypothesis involving the coagulation cascade has been identified as another underlying mechanism initiating thromboembolic events in patients with TTC. Studies showed a significant increase in coagulation factors such as von Willebrand factor, prothrombin, and fibrinogen, collectively known as the acute phase proteins.[39] This phenomenon has also been reported in patients with ACS and further diagnostic tools should be considered in patients with TTC, especially those with markedly elevated D-dimer levels.

A therapeutic anticoagulation dose is recommended for patients with TTC complicated with the formation of a ventricular thrombus. In patients with TTC who present with chest pain and are suspected of having an ACS, there is a distinct possibility that anticoagulation would be prescribed upon first medical assessment, and this could potentially decrease the rate of thrombus formation and embolic events in TTC.

SUMMARY

Thromboembolic events such as ventricular thrombus formation, stroke, and peripheral embolization are important complications of TTC. It can occur both at initial presentation or at any time later during the disease course. Nevertheless, the risk of thromboembolic events in TTC may be underestimated. This may be partly owing to the time delay involved in obtaining a repeat echocardiographic assessment, frequency of tests and also operator skills. A vital component of the diagnostic and disease management chain is the physicians experience treating patients with TTC, the involvement of an interdisciplinary team, and the streamlined treatment of such thromboembolic events on a patient individualized basis (**Fig. 3**). Close follow-up of all patients with TTC presenting with thromboembolic complications is necessary so as to document any change in LV function,

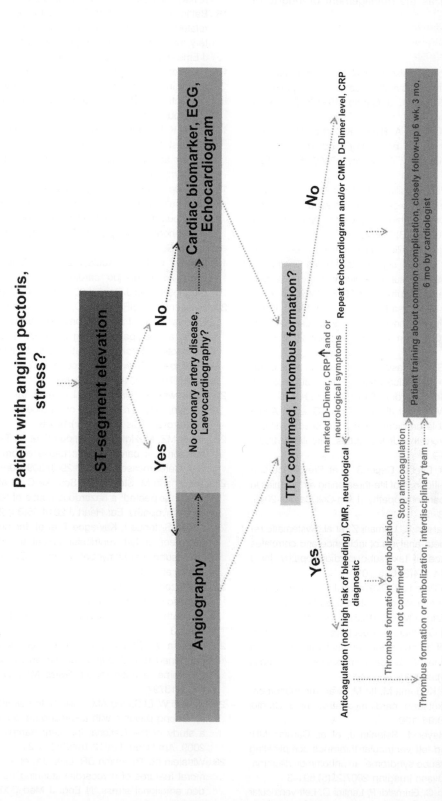

Fig. 3. Proposal of simplified algorithm in patients with takotsubo cardiomyopathy at risk of thromboembolic events. CMR, cardiac MRI; CRP, C-reactive protein; ECG, electrocardiograph.

observe recurrence of TTC, and thrombosis resolution, as well as the management of long-term therapy.

REFERENCES

1. Dote K, Sato H, Tateishi H, et al. Myocardial stunning due to simultaneous multivessel coronary spasms: a review of 5 cases. J Cardiol 1991;21(2):203–14 [in Japanese].

2. Elesber A, Lerman A, Bybee KA, et al. Myocardial perfusion in apical ballooning syndrome correlate of myocardial injury. Am Heart J 2006;152(3). 469. e9-e.13.

3. Haghi D, Papavassiliu T, Fluchter S, et al. Variant form of the acute apical ballooning syndrome (takotsubo cardiomyopathy): observations on a novel entity. Heart 2006;92(3):392–4.

4. Haghi D, Papavassiliu T, Heggemann F, et al. Incidence and clinical significance of left ventricular thrombus in tako-tsubo cardiomyopathy assessed with echocardiography. QJM 2008;101(5):381–6.

5. Madhavan M, Prasad A. Proposed Mayo Clinic criteria for the diagnosis of Tako-Tsubo cardiomyopathy and long-term prognosis. Herz 2010;35(4): 240–3.

6. Schneider B, Athanasiadis A, Schwab J, et al. Complications in the clinical course of tako-tsubo cardiomyopathy. Int J Cardiol 2014;176(1):199–205.

7. Sharkey SW, Lesser JR, Zenovich AG, et al. Acute and reversible cardiomyopathy provoked by stress in women from the United States. Circulation 2005; 111(4):472–9.

8. Stiermaier T, Eitel C, Denef S, et al. Prevalence and clinical significance of life-threatening arrhythmias in takotsubo cardiomyopathy. J Am Coll Cardiol 2015; 65(19):2148–50.

9. Singh K, Carson K, Usmani Z, et al. Systematic review and meta-analysis of incidence and correlates of recurrence of takotsubo cardiomyopathy. Int J Cardiol 2014;174(3):696–701.

10. Templin C, Ghadri JR, Diekmann J, et al. Clinical features and outcomes of takotsubo (stress) cardiomyopathy. N Engl J Med 2015;373(10):929–38.

11. Korosoglou G, Haars A, Kuecherer H, et al. Prompt resolution of an apical left ventricular thrombus in a patient with takotsubo cardiomyopathy. Int J Cardiol 2007;116(3):e88–91.

12. Mitsuma W, Kodama M, Ito M, et al. Thromboembolism in Takotsubo cardiomyopathy. Int J Cardiol 2010;139(1):98–100.

13. Singh V, Mayer T, Salanitri J, et al. Cardiac MRI documented left ventricular thrombus complicating acute Takotsubo syndrome: an uncommon dilemma. Int J Cardiovasc Imaging 2007;23(5):591–3.

14. de Gregorio C, Grimaldi P, Lentini C. Left ventricular thrombus formation and cardioembolic complications in patients with Takotsubo-like syndrome: a systematic review. Int J Cardiol 2008;131(1):18–24.

15. Battimelli A, Polito MV, Di Maio M, et al. Stress-related cardiomyopathy, ventricular dysfunction, artery thrombosis: a hidden pheochromocytoma. Am J Emerg Med 2014;32(3). 286.e5-e9.

16. de Gregorio C, Cento D, Di Bella G, et al. Minor stroke in a Takotsubo-like syndrome: a rare clinical presentation due to transient left ventricular thrombus. Int J Cardiol 2008;130(2):e78–80.

17. Ouchi K, Nakamura F, Ikutomi M, et al. Usefulness of contrast computed tomography to detect left ventricular apical thrombus associated with takotsubo cardiomyopathy. Heart Vessels 2016;31(5):822–7.

18. Mrdovic I, Perunicic J, Asanin M, et al. Transient left ventricular apical ballooning complicated by a mural thrombus and outflow tract obstruction in a patient with pheochromocytoma. Tex Heart Inst J 2008; 35(4):480–2.

19. Hrymak C, Liu S, Koulack J, et al. Embolus from probable Takotsubo cardiomyopathy: a bedside diagnosis. Can J Cardiol 2014;30(12). 1732.e9-e11.

20. Gnanenthiran SR, Amos D, Kamaladasa K, et al. Occlusive radial artery thrombosis following severe radial artery spasm during coronary angiography in Takotsubo Cardiomyopathy: should this access route be avoided in this condition? Int J Cardiol 2015;179:38–9.

21. Grabowski A, Kilian J, Strank C, et al. Takotsubo cardiomyopathy–a rare cause of cardioembolic stroke. Cerebrovasc Dis 2007;24(1):146–8.

22. Jabiri MZ, Mazighi M, Meimoun P, et al. Tako-tsubo syndrome: a cardioembolic cause of brain infarction. Cerebrovasc Dis 2010;29(3):309–10.

23. Koopmann M, Stepper W, Schulke C, et al. Expect the (un)expected: a hazardous cause of tako-tsubo cardiomyopathy. Eur Heart J 2014;35(34):2272.

24. Kurisu S, Inoue I, Kawagoe T, et al. Incidence and treatment of left ventricular apical thrombosis in Tako-tsubo cardiomyopathy. Int J Cardiol 2011; 146(3):e58–60.

25. Matsuzono K, Ikeda Y, Deguchi S, et al. Cerebral embolic stroke after disappearing takotsubo cardiomyopathy. J Stroke Cerebrovasc Dis 2013;22(8): e682–3.

26. Valbusa A, Paganini M, Secchi G, et al. What happened to a thrombus during apical ballooning syndrome: a case report. Swiss Med Wkly 2013; 143:w13797.

27. Brinjikji W, El-Sayed AM, Salka S. In-hospital mortality among patients with takotsubo cardiomyopathy: a study of the National Inpatient Sample 2008 to 2009. Am Heart J 2012;164(2):215–21.

28. Wittstein IS, Thiemann DR, Lima JA, et al. Neurohumoral features of myocardial stunning due to sudden emotional stress. N Engl J Med 2005;352(6): 539–48.

29. Kurisu S, Inoue I, Kawagoe T. Conditions associated with left ventricular apical ballooning. Clin Cardiol 2010;33(6):E123–4.

30. Tsuchihashi K, Ueshima K, Uchida T, et al. Transient left ventricular apical ballooning without coronary artery stenosis: a novel heart syndrome mimicking acute myocardial infarction. Angina Pectoris-Myocardial Infarction Investigations in Japan. J Am Coll Cardiol 2001;38(1):11–8.

31. Nihoyannopoulos P, Smith GC, Maseri A, et al. The natural history of left ventricular thrombus in myocardial infarction: a rationale in support of masterly inactivity. J Am Coll Cardiol 1989;14(4):903–11.

32. Roifman I, Connelly KA, Wright GA, et al. Echocardiography vs. cardiac magnetic resonance imaging for the diagnosis of left ventricular thrombus: a systematic review. Can J Cardiol 2015;31(6):785–91.

33. Mahmood MM, Mahmood S. Unusual echocardiographic appearance of left ventricular thrombi in a patient with dilated cardiomyopathy. BMJ Case Rep 2014;2014 [pii:bcr2014204416].

34. Aryal MR, Badal M, Giri S, et al. Left ventricular non-compaction presenting with heart failure and intramural thrombus. BMJ Case Rep 2013;2013 [pii: bcr2013009757].

35. Aguilar JA, Summerson C. Intracardiac thrombus in antiphospholipid antibody syndrome. J Am Soc Echocardiogr 2000;13(9):873–5.

36. Barjatiya MK, Shah NK, Kothari SS, et al. Spontaneous left ventricle cavity thrombus in a patient of systemic lupus erythematosus. J Assoc Physicians India 1992;40(3):195–6.

37. Ejima J, Ohmura I, Kaji Y, et al. Diffuse endocardial thrombus in left ventricle associated with a case of hypereosinophilic syndrome. Jpn Heart J 1991; 32(2):267–72.

38. Vanhaleweyk G, el-Ramahi KM, Hazmi M, et al. Right atrial, right ventricular and left ventricular thrombi in (incomplete) Behcet's disease. Eur Heart J 1990; 11(10):957–9.

39. Parkkonen O, Mustonen P, Puurunen M, et al. Coagulation changes in takotsubo cardiomyopathy support acute phase reaction and catecholamine excess, but not thrombus production. Int J Cardiol 2014;177(3):1063–5.

40. Cecchi E, Parodi G, Fatucchi S, et al. Prevalence of thrombophilic disorders in takotsubo patients: the (ThROmbophylia in TAkotsubo cardiomyopathy) TROTA study. Clin Res Cardiol 2016. [Epub ahead of print].

41. Davidsen C, Larsen TH, Gerdts E, et al. Giant right ventricular outflow tract thrombus in hereditary spherocytosis: a case report. Thromb J 2016;14:9.

42. Rinuncini M, Zuin M, Scaranello F, et al. Differentiation of cardiac thrombus from cardiac tumor combining cardiac MRI and 18F-FDG-PET/CT Imaging. Int J Cardiol 2016;212:94–6.

43. Weinsaft JW, Kim HW, Crowley AL, et al. LV thrombus detection by routine echocardiography: insights into performance characteristics using delayed enhancement CMR. JACC Cardiovasc Imaging 2011;4(7):702–12.

44. Powers WJ, Derdeyn CP, Biller J, et al. 2015 American Heart Association/American Stroke Association Focused Update of the 2013 guidelines for the early management of patients with acute ischemic stroke regarding endovascular treatment: a guideline for healthcare professionals from the American Heart Association/American Stroke Association. Stroke 2015;46(10):3020–35.

45. de Gregorio C, Ando G. A rare cause of Takotsubo cardiomyopathy related left ventricular apical thrombus requiring surgery. Heart Lung Circ 2012; 21(4):251.

46. Seitz MJ, McLeod MK, O'Keefe MD, et al. A rare cause of Takotsubo cardiomyopathy related left ventricular apical thrombus requiring surgery. Heart Lung Circ 2012;21(4):245–6.

47. Figueredo VM, Gupta S. Embolic complication of Tako-Tsubo cardiomyopathy. QJM 2009;102(11): 820–2.

48. Kimura K, Tanabe-Hayashi Y, Noma S, et al. Images in cardiovascular medicine. Rapid formation of left ventricular giant thrombus with Takotsubo cardiomyopathy. Circulation 2007;115(23): e620–1.

49. Sasaki N, Kinugawa T, Yamawaki M, et al. Transient left ventricular apical ballooning in a patient with bicuspid aortic valve created a left ventricular thrombus leading to acute renal infarction. Circ J 2004;68(11):1081–3.

50. Abe Y, Kondo M, Matsuoka R, et al. Assessment of clinical features in transient left ventricular apical ballooning. J Am Coll Cardiol 2003;41(5):737–42.

51. Maron BJ, Towbin JA, Thiene G, et al. Contemporary definitions and classification of the cardiomyopathies: an American Heart Association Scientific Statement from the Council on Clinical Cardiology, Heart Failure and Transplantation Committee; Quality of Care and Outcomes Research and Functional Genomics and Translational Biology Interdisciplinary Working Groups; and Council on Epidemiology and Prevention. Circulation 2006;113(14): 1807–16.

52. Gianni M, Dentali F, Grandi AM, et al. Apical ballooning syndrome or takotsubo cardiomyopathy: a systematic review. Eur Heart J 2006;27(13): 1523–9.

53. Bybee KA, Prasad A. Stress-related cardiomyopathy syndromes. Circulation 2008;118(4):397–409.

54. de Gregorio C. Cardioembolic outcomes in stress-related cardiomyopathy complicated by ventricular thrombus: a systematic review of 26 clinical studies. Int J Cardiol 2010;141(1):11–7.

55. Vaitkus PT, Barnathan ES. Embolic potential, prevention and management of mural thrombus complicating anterior myocardial infarction: a meta-analysis. J Am Coll Cardiol 1993;22(4):1004–9.

56. Greaves SC, Zhi G, Lee RT, et al. Incidence and natural history of left ventricular thrombus following anterior wall acute myocardial infarction. Am J Cardiol 1997;80(4):442–8.

57. Bybee KA, Prasad A, Barsness GW, et al. Clinical characteristics and thrombolysis in myocardial infarction frame counts in women with transient left ventricular apical ballooning syndrome. Am J Cardiol 2004;94(3):343–6.

58. Anzai T, Yoshikawa T, Kaneko H, et al. Association between serum C-reactive protein elevation and left ventricular thrombus formation after first anterior myocardial infarction. Chest 2004;125(2):384–9.

59. Shin SN, Yun KH, Ko JS, et al. Left ventricular thrombus associated with takotsubo cardiomyopathy: a cardioembolic cause of cerebral infarction. J Cardiovasc Ultrasound 2011;19(3):152–5.

60. Hessel EA 2nd. The brain and the heart. Anesth Analg 2006;103(3):522–6.

61. Loh E, Sutton MS, Wun CC, et al. Ventricular dysfunction and the risk of stroke after myocardial infarction. N Engl J Med 1997;336(4):251–7.

Challenges of Chronic Cardiac Problems in Survivors of Takotsubo Syndrome

Andrew C. Morley-Smith, MA, MB BChir, MRCP[a,b],
Alexander R. Lyon, MA, BM BCh, PhD, FRCP[a,b,*]

KEYWORDS

- Takotsubo • Persistent • Recurrence • Psychology

KEY POINTS

- Takotsubo syndrome (TSS) has to date been seen as a fully reversible and therefore benign form of cardiac dysfunction, but there is increasing evidence that disputes this.
- After an acute episode of TSS, many patients continue to experience a significant cardiovascular and psychological symptom burden that impairs quality of life.
- Converging evidence from imaging, biomarker, and histologic studies suggests that there is persistent cardiac dysfunction that may be related to chronic postinflammatory changes within the myocardium.
- Current data on long-term outcome in TSS is largely confined to observational registry and cohort studies, often without control data, and further work is needed to understand prognosis and optimal therapeutic strategy after an acute episode of TSS.
- The Takotsubo community has made enormous progress over the past 10 years in increasing recognition of TSS in the acute presentation and showing that it is not rare, and the next step is continuing this good practice into chronic care and showing that it is not always benign.

INTRODUCTION

The characteristics of Takotsubo syndrome (TTS) in the acute phase are well described and reviewed in depth in other articles in this issue and elsewhere,[1,2] most recently in a position statement[3] from the Heart Failure Association of the European Society of Cardiology (ESC). Most episodes of TTS originate in a catecholamine surge triggered by physical or emotional stress. This causes an inflammatory catecholaminergic myocarditis with the characteristic clinical findings of cardiac chest pain and dyspnea accompanied by regional wall motion abnormality (RWMA), most frequently apical hypokinesia with basal hypercontractility, in the absence of coronary artery disease that could explain the RWMA.

Disclosures and Conflicts: None to declare.
Funding Statement: A.C. Morley-Smith is a British Heart Foundation Clinical Research Training Fellow (FS/13/34/30173) and A.R. Lyon is a British Heart Foundation Intermediate Clinical Research Fellow (FS/11/67/28954). Both authors are supported by the National Institute for Health Research Cardiovascular Biomedical Research Unit at Royal Brompton & Harefield NHS Foundation Trust.
[a] National Institute for Health Research Cardiovascular Biomedical Research Unit, Royal Brompton & Harefield NHS Foundation Trust, National Heart & Lung Institute, Imperial College London, London, UK; [b] Royal Brompton Hospital, Sydney Street, London SW3 6NP, UK
* Corresponding author. Royal Brompton Hospital, Sydney Street, London SW3 6NP, UK
E-mail address: A.Lyon@imperial.ac.uk

Heart Failure Clin 12 (2016) 551–557
http://dx.doi.org/10.1016/j.hfc.2016.06.006

heartfailure.theclinics.com

Historically TTS has been viewed as fully reversible, such that, whatever the burden of acute duress, cardiac function is assessed as normal at 3 month follow-up, and most patients will be reassured and discharged from cardiac services.

However, there is increasing evidence that the evolution of TTS is not as benign or straightforward as once thought. The pattern and degree of hypokinesia, and the extent to which this causes functional impairment, are highly variable. It is becoming increasingly apparent that most patients (many remaining undiagnosed) have persisting microscopic cardiac dysfunction that may never be apparent clinically, but some TTS survivors experience symptoms. Some have major adverse cardiac events, and some have recurrence of TTS. Recurrence of TTS is one of the most troublesome challenges in the post-TTS cohort, as patients re-enter the high risk phase with acute heart failure, pulmonary edema, arrhythmia, cardiogenic shock, or death. Complications are twice as likely in patients over 75 years old,[4] and recent data from the SWEDEHEART (Swedish Web-system for Enhancement and Development of Evidence-based care in Heart disease Evaluated According to Recommended Therapies) registry suggests TTS patients are three times more likely than NSTEMI (Non ST elevation myocardial infarction) patients to develop to cardiogenic shock.[5] The recent ESC position statement proposes a scoring system whereby high-risk patients may be identified early on clinical grounds.[3]

Increasing recognition of long-term morbidity in the form of ongoing symptoms and syndrome recurrence is important for the clinical community. This parallels the increasing recognition across cardiology that resolution of RWMA and return to normal left ventricular ejection fraction (LVEF) does not necessarily indicate complete cardiac recovery, with more subtle markers based on deformation imaging suggesting otherwise. The spectrum of acute presentation in TTS may reflect varying severity of catecholaminergic myocarditis, in turn paralleled by a spectrum of permanent myocardial damage, varying from minimal diffuse fibrosis to significant ongoing chronic inflammation or larger areas of focal scar. The latter group of patients may be susceptible to persistent cardiac symptoms, recurrence of TTS, or premature death.

PERSISTENT CLINICAL PROBLEMS AND PROGNOSIS

Even without full recurrence of TTS, patients can have significant ongoing symptoms. In a TTS follow-up clinic, the predominant postacute complaints are exertional chest pain, dyspnea, palpitations, and general fatigue, and together these can cause significant functional impairment. In the absence of occlusive coronary disease and recovery of LVEF, patients are frequently informed their symptoms may be secondary to psychological factors, given the writ that TTS resolves completely. However this is not the case, and frequently they have true cardiac origin.

The frequency of postacute symptoms is difficult to estimate, as studies to date have typically not reported follow-up data or grouped symptoms together as major adverse cardiovascular events (MACE) occurring after discharge from the hospital. The rate of late MACE varies between studies. Some of this variability may be due to differing predisposition and differing use of heart failure therapies in the postacute phase. The largest recent cohort with long-term data found MACE occurring at 9.9% per patient–year, and saw improved survival 1 year after the acute TTS episode in patients discharged on an angiotensin converting enzyme ACE inhibitor, although there was no improvement with beta blockade.[6] In this cohort, males had a higher rate of chronic complications, though this may reflect their greater preponderance to cardiovascular risk and superadded effects on the cardiovascular system.

The rate of TTS recurrence has varied from 0% to 22% in different cohorts.[7,8] However, a larger contemporary cohort showed recurrence of 1.8% per patient–year, representing just 57 recurrences in the 1750 TTS patients studied (3%), occurring 25 days to 9.2 years from the first event.[6] This supports Singh and colleagues'[8] meta-analysis in 2014, which showed incidence of recurrence at 1.5% per year. There are some data that identify right ventricular (RV) involvement and corrected QT interval (QTc) duration at initial presentation as predictors of greater long-term morbidity and mortality.[9,10]

Data for long-term outcomes in TTS survivors remains incomplete. As the fields begins to challenge the perception of TTS as a single acute illness, contemporary registries and observational studies are needed to generate long-term follow-up data that could properly address prognosis. Three studies have data available now. Templin and colleagues[6] report all-cause death at 5.6%/year in their cohort over 10 years of follow-up. This is a TTS registry, however, and there is no control group for comparison (**Fig. 1**A). A recent study compared 286 TTS patients with age- and gender-matched STEMI survivors, and found 58% excess mortality in the TTS group (24.7% vs 15.1%, hazard ratio 1.58, 95% confidence

A

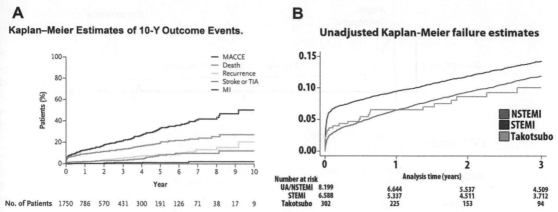

Fig. 1. Kaplan-Meier estimates of long term outcome in TTS. (*A*) There is a significant cardiovascular morbidity burden after an episode of TTS. This single-arm registry study of 1750 patients with TTS found that around half of patients will experience a major adverse cardiovascular event by 10 years (9.9% per patient–year). (*B*) Mortality after TTS is equivalent to that after ST elevation myocardial infarction (STEMI) and non-ST elevation myocardial infarction (NSTEMI). This registry study compared long-term outcomes from TTS, illustrated in this Kaplan-Meier estimate out to 3 years. (*From* [A] Templin C, Ghadri JR, Diekmann J, et al. Clinical Features and outcomes of Takotsubo (stress) cardiomyopathy. N Engl J Med 2015;373(10):936, with permission; and [B] Redfors B, Vedad R, Angeras O, et al. Mortality in Takotsubo syndrome is similar to mortality in myocardial infarction—a report from the SWEDEHEART registry. Int J Cardiol 2015;185:287, with permission.)

interval 1.07–2.33; $P = .02$).[11] Furthermore the SWEDEHEART registry of acute chest pain admissions includes 302 (2%) TTS cases from 15,348 patients, and shows lifetime mortality equivalent between TTS, NSTEMI, and STEMI[5] (**Fig. 1**B). It is unclear from these observational data whether the mortality burden in TTS is caused by long-standing damage from the TTS, or due to the higher preponderance of comorbidities in the TTS group at baseline (both cardiovascular and noncardiovascular comorbidities). This relatively poor prognosis compared with ischemic population is different from common perception.

EVIDENCE FOR PERSISTING CARDIOVASCULAR ABNORMALITIES

There is convergent clinical, circulating biomarker, and imaging evidence that there are persistent myocardial abnormalities after the acute TTS episode (**Fig. 2**).

Left Ventricular Function

Numerous historic studies have reported resolution of LV systolic function after the acute TTS episode, basing this assessment on gross function parameters, in particular LVEF.[3,6,12–15] Gianni and colleagues'[14] systematic review shows LVEF improving from 20% to 49% on admission to 60% to 76% at follow-up, and the recent report from Templin and colleagues[6] confirms this in a more contemporary cohort, with mean LVEF improving from 41.1% (n = 1179) to 59.9%

(n = 290, dropout is loss to follow-up) by 60 days. Some studies have shown recovery of LVEF is delayed in a subset of patients before ultimately returning to normal (5% in 1 study[16]).

However, newer approaches with advanced echocardiography and cardiac magnetic resonance (CMR) imaging techniques have suggested a more subtle long-term deficit in systolic function. Neil and colleagues[17] studied 36 TTS patients and 19 controls out to 3 months after the acute episode. LVEF was significantly reduced acutely (LVEF 52 vs 63%, $P<.01$) and had normalized (LVEF 60%) by 3-month reassessment, but the global longitudinal strain (GLS) assessed by speckle echocardiography was impaired acutely (-12.7 vs -20%, $P<.001$) and remained impaired at 3 months (-17.9%, $P<.01$). Furthermore, the degree of GLS impairment correlates with NT-proBNP and with impaired quality of life on a questionnaire assessment.[17] A small CMR study showed persistent markers of diastolic dysfunction (LV filling rates and left atrial size) despite early resolution of systolic function parameters.[18] Biventricular involvement in the acute presentation carries heightened acute mortality[4] and may bring increased risk of recurrence and long-term morbidity.[9] This may reflect comorbidities predating the TTS and predisposing to biventricular presentation rather than a consequence of the TTS per se.

These data support the hypothesis that LV function does not normalize completely, but remains subtly impaired for several months after the acute presentation.

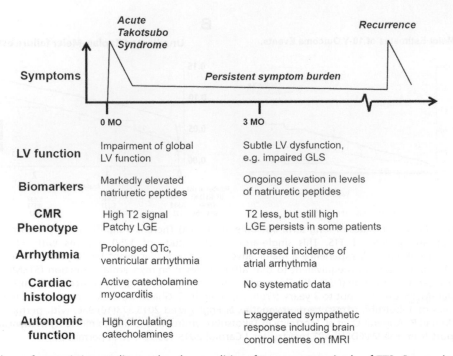

Fig. 2. Evidence for persisting cardiovascular abnormalities after an acute episode of TTS. Converging evidence supports the hypothesis that there is acute catecholaminergic myocarditis in TTS, inflammation that gradually settles over several months after the acute episode. However, in many cases, the myocardial injury does not resolve completely, evidenced by persistent abnormalities of systolic function, abnormal tissue characterization on cardiovascular magnetic resonance, persistent natriuretic peptide elevation, and ongoing propensity to arrhythmia. This results in long-term heightened cardiovascular morbidity and mortality rates equivalent to patients surviving myocardial infarction. See main text for detailed discussion and references.

CMR Myocardial Tissue Characterization

Detailed tissue characterization is a particular strength of CMR over other cardiac imaging modalities and allows one to ascertain potential contributors to this persistent dysfunction. In the acute phase, CMR is an important tool for distinguishing TTS from other pathologies, particularly in excluding myocardial infarction and in discerning TTS from other forms of acute myocarditis.[3]

The archetypal features in the acute phase are RWMA and LV systolic dysfunction alongside myocardial inflammation and/or edema on T2 imaging, and the absence of subendocardial late gadolinium enhancement (LGE) that would be typical of myocardial infarction.[18] T2 imaging demonstrates areas of increased myocardial water content, and in TTS, that might represent inflammation or early fibrosis. LGE is seen in some patients in a patchy subendocardial distribution, which may represent focal replacement fibrosis, and its presence acutely may infer worse long-term prognosis.[19] LGE is not reported in all CMR studies in TTS, and this may relate to different detection thresholds in scanning protocols. One

difficulty is identifying what myocardial pathology these CMR changes actually represent. Both the T2 signal and the patchy LGE could represent myocardial inflammation (leaky capillaries and increased myocardial water content) or fibrosis (expanded extracellular volume), and in fact there may be a continuum of myocardial changes in response to high catecholamine exposure.[20]

In some patients, these abnormalities persist beyond the acute phase, possibly representing longer-term damage and paralleling the more subtle systolic dysfunction seen with strain imaging. Neil and colleagues[21] studied the T2 edema in a prospective cohort of 32 TTS patients, and found it appears in the distribution of the wall motion abnormality, and the degree of edema correlates with acute levels of catecholamines and peak NT-proBNP; by 3 months, the T2-weighted signal had decreased significantly, but not to normal. Evidence from other cohorts of patients with catecholaminergic myocarditis parallels these findings. In a recent study of 60 patients with pheochromocytoma, a catecholamine-releasing tumor, CMR, showed features of catecholaminergic myocarditis in the acute phase (in this study elevated T1 and patchy subendocardial LGE) and chronic changes, probably representing focal or diffuse myocardial fibrosis.[22]

Circulating Biomarkers

Natriuretic peptides are the most useful circulating biomarker in TTS, and elevation of BNP and NT-proBNP during the acute phase is expected and may correlate with hemodynamic parameters,[23–25] although Elsber showed no use for natriuretic peptides or troponin as prognostic markers in TTS.[12] The release of natriuretic peptide is often seen to a greater extent than cardiac troponin, and this can help differentiate TTS from acute coronary syndrome, in particular from true ST elevation infarct when the troponin rises much more than TTS.[23] Moreover, Nguyen and colleagues[25] showed in 56 TTS patients that not only was NT-proBNP markedly elevated in the acute phase, but also that it remained elevated versus controls at 3 months, despite normalization of the acute RWMA. This ongoing release of NT-proBNP supports the notion of ongoing cardiac dysfunction after the acute episode.

Arrhythmia

One study found life-threatening ventricular arrhythmia in 13.5% of patients (24 from 178 consecutive confirmed TTS cases), and found arrhythmia was more prevalent in patients with suggestion of fibrosis on CMR and in patients with longer QTc on admission.[10,26] There is an increased incidence of atrial arrhythmias in patients who have previously experienced an acute TTS episode.[27] Whether this reflects the impact of acute left atrial stretch during the acute phase in the setting of acute LV diastolic pressure elevation remains to be determined, but the persistent natriuretic peptide elevation would be supportive of long-term abnormalities of LV diastolic physiology in the context of recovered LVEF.

Myocardial Histology

One study has systematically studied myocardial histology during the acute episode and in early recovery.[28] The acute changes included vacuole expansion contributing to myocyte hypertrophy, and extracellular matrix expansion with proteins such as collagen. The authors saw a high degree of reversibility of these acute responses to catecholamines. However, although the recovery biopsies were taken after normalization of gross LV function, this was still early in the disease evolution at 12 plus or minus 3 days after presentation, so these do not give a true picture of the long-term histologic recovery. Further tissue

studies could elucidate this and might provide correlation with tissue characterization findings on CMR.

NONCARDIAC PROBLEMS

Psychological health and quality of life are impacted in the long term by TTS. At 1 year after the acute episode, patients show impaired physical quality of life, and when compared directly with patients after myocardial infarction, the same patients showed greater impairments of psychological well being.[29] The degree of residual systolic impairment correlates with quality-of-life impairment.[17] One small study disputed the hypothesis that previous TTS predisposes the myocardium to vulnerability to mental stress,[30] but certainly the possibility of recurrence in an anxious patient can be a serious detriment to psychological health.

Functional brain imaging and studies of the autonomic nervous system have tried to ascertain whether TTS survivors have biological substrate for heightened anxiety. Direct testing of autonomic function was undertaken in TTS survivors versus controls, with both direct physical and central stimuli, and on average 37 months after the acute episode. There was a clear exaggeration of sympathetic stimulation alongside blunted parasympathetic modulation.[31] This is supported by a functional MRI brain imaging study that showed differential activation of autonomic control regions between TTS and control.[32] It is unclear whether these factors serve to precipitate the TTS initially, or whether they represent a postacute phenomenon occurring because of the TTS episode, but in either case, they remain important determinants of long-term psychological health.

Aside from psychological health, there are some reports of association with cancer.[33,34] Whether the association truly exists, and whether the cancer is causative (via a postulated paraneoplastic mechanism) or consequent to the acute TTS, or incidental due to the background risk in postmenopausal women, all remains to be determined.

SUMMARY

TTS has been viewed as an acute cardiac illness without long-term sequelae, but increasing understanding of this patient group is challenging this view. Converging evidence suggests that the acute myocardial insult leaves an ongoing recovery process with subtle impairment to systolic function and important clinical symptoms and complications, including a long-term prognosis equivalent to STEMI.

The next steps are to characterize in more detail the nature and longevity of the chronic myocardial process, its implications for prognosis, and what this means for targeted cardiovascular therapy in TTS. Unanswered questions remain about best management of psychological health in the long term. The TTS field has made enormous progress over the past 10 years in increasing recognition of TTS in the acute presentation and showing that TTS is not rare, and the next step is continuing this good practice into chronic care and showing that TTS is not always benign.

REFERENCES

1. Wright PT, Tranter MH, Morley-Smith AC, et al. Pathophysiology of Takotsubo syndrome: temporal phases of cardiovascular responses to extreme stress. Circ J 2014;78(7):1550–8.
2. Lyon AR, Rees PS, Prasad S, et al. Stress (Takotsubo) cardiomyopathy—a novel pathophysiological hypothesis to explain catecholamine-induced acute myocardial stunning. Nat Clin Pract Cardiovasc Med 2008;5(1):22–9.
3. Lyon AR, Bossone E, Schneider B, et al. Current state of knowledge on Takotsubo syndrome: a position statement from the taskforce on Takotsubo Syndrome of the heart failure association of the European Society of Cardiology. Eur J Heart Fail 2016;18(1):8–27.
4. Citro R, Rigo F, D'Andrea A, et al. Echocardiographic correlates of acute heart failure, cardiogenic shock, and in-hospital mortality in tako-tsubo cardiomyopathy. JACC Cardiovasc Imaging 2014;7(2):119–29.
5. Redfors B, Vedad R, Angeras O, et al. Mortality in takotsubo syndrome is similar to mortality in myocardial infarction—a report from the SWEDEHEART registry. Int J Cardiol 2015;185:282–9.
6. Templin C, Ghadri JR, Diekmann J, et al. Clinical features and outcomes of Takotsubo (stress) cardiomyopathy. N Engl J Med 2015;373(10):929–38.
7. Akashi YJ, Nef HM, Lyon AR. Epidemiology and pathophysiology of Takotsubo syndrome. Nat Rev Cardiol 2015;12(7):387–97.
8. Singh K, Carson K, Usmani Z, et al. Systematic review and meta-analysis of incidence and correlates of recurrence of Takotsubo cardiomyopathy. Int J Cardiol 2014;174(3):696–701.
9. Kagiyama N, Okura H, Tamada T, et al. Impact of right ventricular involvement on the prognosis of Takotsubo cardiomyopathy. Eur Heart J Cardiovasc Imaging 2016;17(2):210–6.
10. Gopalakrishnan M, Hassan A, Villines D, et al. Predictors of short- and long-term outcomes of Takotsubo cardiomyopathy. Am J Cardiol 2015;116(10):1586–90.
11. Stiermaier T, Moeller C, Oehler K, et al. Long-term excess mortality in Takotsubo cardiomyopathy: predictors, causes and clinical consequences. Eur J Heart Fail 2016;18(6):650–6.
12. Elesber AA, Prasad A, Lennon RJ, et al. Four-year recurrence rate and prognosis of the apical ballooning syndrome. J Am Coll Cardiol 2007;50(5):448–52.
13. Eitel I, von Knobelsdorff-Brenkenhoff F, Bernhardt P, et al. Clinical characteristics and cardiovascular magnetic resonance findings in stress (Takotsubo) cardiomyopathy. JAMA 2011;306(3):277–86.
14. Gianni M, Dentali F, Grandi AM, et al. Apical ballooning syndrome or Takotsubo cardiomyopathy: a systematic review. Eur Heart J 2006;27(13):1523–9.
15. Morley-Smith AC, Lyon AR, Omerovic E. Takotsubo cardiomyopathy. Br J Hosp Med (Lond) 2013;74(2):96–103.
16. Sharkey SW, Windenburg DC, Lesser JR, et al. Natural history and expansive clinical profile of stress (Takotsubo) cardiomyopathy. J Am Coll Cardiol 2010;55(4):333–41.
17. Neil CJ, Nguyen TH, Singh K, et al. Relation of delayed recovery of myocardial function after Takotsubo cardiomyopathy to subsequent quality of life. Am J Cardiol 2015;115(8):1085–9.
18. Ahtarovski KA, Iversen KK, Christensen TE, et al. Takotsubo cardiomyopathy, a two-stage recovery of left ventricular systolic and diastolic function as determined by cardiac magnetic resonance imaging. Eur Heart J Cardiovasc Imaging 2014;15(8):855–62.
19. Naruse Y, Sato A, Kasahara K, et al. The clinical impact of late gadolinium enhancement in Takotsubo cardiomyopathy: serial analysis of cardiovascular magnetic resonance images. J Cardiovasc Magn Reson 2011;13:67.
20. Morley-Smith AC, Lyon AR. Stressing the importance of cardiac assessment in pheochromocytoma. J Am Coll Cardiol 2016;67(20):2375–7.
21. Neil C, Nguyen TH, Kucia A, et al. Slowly resolving global myocardial inflammation/oedema in Tako-Tsubo cardiomyopathy: evidence from T2-weighted cardiac MRI. Heart 2012;98(17):1278–84.
22. Ferreira VM, Marcelino M, Piechnik SK, et al. Pheochromocytoma is characterized by catecholamine-mediated myocarditis, focal and diffuse myocardial fibrosis, and myocardial dysfunction. J Am Coll Cardiol 2016;67(20):2364–74.
23. Madhavan M, Borlaug BA, Lerman A, et al. Stress hormone and circulating biomarker profile of apical ballooning syndrome (Takotsubo cardiomyopathy): insights into the clinical significance of B-type natriuretic peptide and troponin levels. Heart 2009;95(17):1436–41.

24. Wittstein IS, Thiemann DR, Lima JA, et al. Neurohumoral features of myocardial stunning due to sudden emotional stress. N Engl J Med 2005;352(6):539–48.

25. Nguyen TH, Neil CJ, Sverdlov AL, et al. N-terminal pro-brain natriuretic protein levels in Takotsubo cardiomyopathy. Am J Cardiol 2011;108(9):1316–21.

26. Stiermaier T, Eitel C, Denef S, et al. Prevalence and clinical significance of life-threatening arrhythmias in Takotsubo cardiomyopathy. J Am Coll Cardiol 2015;65(19):2148–50.

27. Valbusa A, Abbadessa F, Giachero C, et al. Long-term follow-up of Takotsubo-like syndrome: a retrospective study of 22 cases. J Cardiovasc Med (Hagerstown) 2008;9(8):805–9.

28. Nef HM, Mollmann H, Kostin S, et al. Takotsubo cardiomyopathy: intraindividual structural analysis in the acute phase and after functional recovery. Eur Heart J 2007;28(20):2456–64.

29. Compare A, Grossi E, Bigi R, et al. Stress-induced cardiomyopathy and psychological wellbeing 1 year after an acute event. J Clin Psychol Med Settings 2014;21(1):81–91.

30. Collste O, Tornvall P, Sundin O, et al. No myocardial vulnerability to mental stress in Takotsubo stress cardiomyopathy. PLoS One 2014;9(4):e93697.

31. Norcliffe-Kaufmann L, Kaufmann H, Martinez J, et al. Autonomic findings in Takotsubo cardiomyopathy. Am J Cardiol 2016;117(2):206–13.

32. Pereira VH, Marques P, Magalhaes R, et al. Central autonomic nervous system response to autonomic challenges is altered in patients with a previous episode of Takotsubo cardiomyopathy. Eur Heart J Acute Cardiovasc Care 2016;5(2):152–63.

33. El-Sayed AM, Brinjikji W, Salka S. Demographic and co-morbid predictors of stress (Takotsubo) cardiomyopathy. Am J Cardiol 2012;110(9):1368–72.

34. Burgdorf C, Kurowski V, Bonnemeier H, et al. Long-term prognosis of the transient left ventricular dysfunction syndrome (Takotsubo cardiomyopathy): focus on malignancies. Eur J Heart Fail 2008;10(10):1015–9.

Contemporary Imaging in Takotsubo Syndrome

Rodolfo Citro, MD, PhD[a],*, Gianluca Pontone, MD, PhD[b], Leonardo Pace, MD[c],
Concetta Zito, MD, PhD[d], Angelo Silverio, MD[a], Eduardo Bossone, PhD, FCCP, FESC, FACC[a],
Federico Piscione, MD[a,c]

KEYWORDS

- Takotsubo syndrome • Stress cardiomyopathy • Apical ballooning syndrome • Echocardiography
- Cardiac magnetic resonance • Coronary computed tomography angiography
- Single photon emission computed tomography • Positron emission tomography

KEY POINTS

- Transthoracic echocardiography is the first-line noninvasive imaging modality for the early evaluation of patients with suspected Takotsubo syndrome and for monitoring myocardial function and hemodynamic conditions during the acute phase. However, in recent years, cardiac magnetic resonance and coronary computed tomography angiography have been assuming an emerging role to confirm diagnosis because of their unique ability to obtain information about myocardial tissue characterization and coronary artery patency.
- Patients with Takotsubo syndrome typically show the apical ballooning pattern characterized by akinesia or dyskinesia of the apical and midventricular segments of the left ventricle, and hyperkinesia of the base. However, several variant morphologies, such as midventricular, basal, inverted or even focal forms, have also been described.
- A circumferential pattern of regional wall motion abnormalities beyond the territory of a single coronary artery distribution is a distinctive marker of Takotsubo syndrome that can be easily appreciated with both echocardiography and cardiac magnetic resonance.
- Owing to the possibility of detecting mechanical complications, including intraventricular pressure gradients, reversible functional mitral regurgitation, right ventricular involvement, intraventricular thrombi, and pericardial effusion, echocardiography is useful not only for diagnostic purposes but also for risk stratification.
- Molecular imaging has emerged in the last few years for the possibility of assessing functional and molecular processes.

INTRODUCTION

The diagnosis of Takotsubo syndrome (TTS) is based on a series of criteria, including medical history and clinical and instrumental findings.[1–3] In the last decades, the development of sophisticated noninvasive imaging modalities has provided a unique opportunity to improve knowledge about this intriguing syndrome.[1–3]

Taking into account the large amount of data available in the literature on TTS, this article will

No commercial or financial conflicts of interest and any funding sources to declare.
a Department of Cardiology, University Hospital "San Giovanni di Dio e Ruggi d'Aragona," Heart Tower Room 810, Largo Città di Ippocrate, Salerno 84131, Italy; b Centro Cardiolgico Monzino, IRCCS, Via Carlo Parea 4, 20138, Milan, Italy; c Department of Medicine and Surgery, Schola Medica Salernitana, University of Salerno, Via Salvador Allende, 84081 Baronissi (Salerno), Italy; d Cardiology, Department of Clinical and Experimental Medicine, University of Messina, Piazza Pugliatti 1, 98122 Messina, Italy
* Corresponding author. University Hospital "San Giovanni di Dio e Ruggi d'Aragona", Heart Tower Room 810, Largo Città di Ippocrate, Salerno 84131, Italy.
E-mail address: rodolfocitro@gmail.com

review the main noninvasive imaging techniques and their clinical application for diagnostic work-up, risk stratification, and monitoring follow-up.

ECHOCARDIOGRAPHY

Owing to its widespread availability and bedside feasibility even in the acute care setting, transthoracic echocardiography (TTE) is the first-line noninvasive imaging modality for the evaluation of patients with suspected TTS for diagnostic and prognostic stratification and monitoring myocardial function recovery during follow-up.

DIAGNOSTIC MARKERS
Regional Wall Motion Abnormalities

Regional wall motion abnormalities (WMAs) have a typical distribution in patients with TTS. Topography of WMA tends to involve the apical and mid-ventricular myocardial segments circumferentially beyond the territory of a single coronary artery distribution (**Fig. 1**).[1–3] Such circumferential pattern has been considered as a distinctive feature of TTS and included in the differential diagnosis between TTS and acute coronary syndrome.[1] Global longitudinal strain (GLS) can be used to assess regional myocardial function in various conditions, and it has been found to have high sensitivity for the diagnosis of patients with acute myocardial infarctions (AMIs).[4–7] In a recent case series, a characteristic pattern in the GLS polar map of TTS patients that is not typical of any specific coronary distribution has been appreciated; this pattern affects only the apical segments, similar to the known image of the evil eye (**Fig. 2**).[8] This pattern is usually observed in the acute phase of TTS, and its recognition may serve as a potential clinical application in those cases with the classic apical ballooning.[8] Of note, in different studies

comparing regional and global alterations of systolic function in TTS versus AMI, it has been demonstrated that in TTS, radial strain is reduced along the entire mid-left ventricular (LV) circumference, and not only in the anterior and anteroseptal wall as in AMI.[9–11] Moreover, in patients with classical TTS, GLS decreased from base ($-15.9 + 6.1\%$) to apex ($-1.7 + 7.6$, $P<.001$) at baseline, with a significant apex-to-base gradient, indicating more severe involvement of the apex.[9] However, despite the perception of basal hypercontractility in TTS, often longitudinal strain of the LV base is also diminished during the acute phase. This reduction of basal strain may be related, in part, to sympathetically mediated myocardial stunning, which may also involve the basal myocardium. It is also conceivable that, similar to what has been observed in patients with AMI, remote loading effects of dysfunctional segments, changes in LV geometry with subsequent increase of wall stress in nonaffected myocardium, and tethering of the basal segments by dysfunctional segments all play a contributory role to the observed decrease in basal longitudinal strain.[9] It has also been demonstrated that both global and regional strain pattern alterations occurring in the acute phase of the disease improve at early follow-up (34 ± 16 days).[9] In particular, average longitudinal and radial strains that were $-10.6 + 5.5\%$ and $20.1 + 17.3\%$, respectively, on hospital admission, improved to $-17.6 + 3.0\%$, and $50.2 + 17.0\%$, respectively (all $P<.001$) during follow-up.[9] The main differences between echocardiographic findings in TTS versus AMI are summarized in **Table 1**.

Morphologic Patterns

According to the localization of WMA, standard TTE allows one to detect different LV morphologic

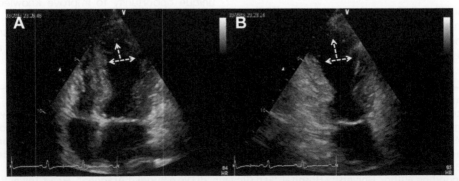

Fig. 1. TTE 4-chamber view (*A*) and 2-chamber view (*B*) of a middle-aged postmenopausal woman admitted to the coronary care unit for chest pain. Note the typical distribution of WMA involving the middle and apical segments of the whole left ventricle (circumferential pattern, see *dotted arrows*), known as apical ballooning associated with hypercontractility of the base.

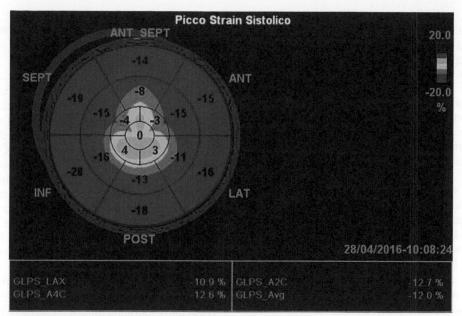

Fig. 2. An example of a polar map of GLS in a patient with TTS. The typical pattern of reduced longitudinal deformation at the apex with significant involvement also of all mid segments (circumferential pattern) and anterior and anteroseptal segments of the LV base can be appreciated. This pattern is markedly different from the recognized pattern in anterior AMI.

Table 1
Main echocardiographic findings in patients with Takotsubo syndrome versus acute coronary syndrome at presentation

	TTS	ACS
LV systolic function	Marked reduction in LV EF on admission with improvement at short term	Varies depending on infarct area
LV wall motion abnormalities	Independent of the distribution of epicardial coronary artery (circumferential pattern) Apical ballooning Variant form: Midventricular ballooning Inverted TTS	Involves myocardial segments supplied by the culprit coronary artery
RV involvement	Reverse McConnell sign (biventricular ballooning)	Dilated with impaired systolic function in ACS secondary to proximal RCA occlusion
Speckle-tracking	Circumferential impairment of LV longitudinal and radial strain	Impaired strain in the myocardial segments supplied by the culprit coronary artery
Coronary flow	Preserved distally to the coronary artery Coronary flow reserve is impaired in the acute phase	Reduced or absent distally to the culprit coronary artery
Additional findings and complications	LVOTO Reversible mitral regurgitation Apical thrombi	Cardiac rupture Mitral regurgitation Apical thrombi Interventricular septum rupture Pericardial effusion

patterns.[12–14] Typically, TTS is characterized by apical ballooning in about 70% to 80% of cases (involving the apical and midventricular segments, which appear akinetic or dyskinetic, in contrast to the basal segments, which are hyperkinetic) (see **Fig. 1**).[14,15] However, several variant forms, such as midventricular or inverted TTS, have also been described.[2] Midventricular TTS is characterized by akinesis of the midventricular segments, mild hypokinesis, or normal contraction of the apical segments and hypercontractility of the base (**Fig. 3**).[2] Inverted TTS is characterized by 2 different forms; the first one is defined as apical sparing with preserved apical function and severe hypokinesis of the remaining walls, and the second one is defined as basal or reverse TTS, with hypokinesis confined to the basal segments (see **Fig. 3**).[2] Nevertheless, no differences have been reported among the several forms of TTS in LV function recovery at early and late follow-up. TTE in the acute phase is also fundamental to identify the rare focal forms that are associated with limited and rapidly reversible WMA that cannot be detected over the first hours or days.[14] Recently, the introduction of real time 3-dimensional echocardiography (RT-3DE) in daily practice, although challenging to perform in the acute care setting, appeared helpful to define LV morphology and systolic function in TTS patients.[2,16–19]

Left Ventricular Systolic Function

LV ejection fraction (EF) is reduced in TTS patients in the acute phase and recovers after resolution of myocardial stunning.[20,21] The degree of EF decrease varies according to the severity of myocardial impairment, presence of comorbidities, and age.[22,23] Generally, a discrepancy between the magnitude of myocardial dysfunction and the modest increment in troponin levels as well as in electrocardiographic changes of ST-T on admission can be appreciated.[2]

Coronary Flow Reserve

The visualization of flow in the distal part of the left anterior descending coronary artery (LAD) is a serendipitous finding in the context of extensive akinesia of the LV apex, reinforcing the diagnostic suspicion of TTS (**Fig. 4**). Nevertheless, in stable patients with typical TTS, in whom no underlying significant coronary narrowing is expected, noninvasive coronary flow reserve (CFR) measured using intravenous vasodilators (eg, adenosine or dipyridamole) in the distal LAD and the posterior descending artery is impaired during the acute phase of the disease and improves significantly by nearly 40% at follow-up.[24–28]

Of note, there is a reversible dysfunction of coronary microcirculation in regions with and without WMA demonstrating diffuse impairment of the coronary microcirculation, as also documented with other invasive techniques.[29] The recovery of CFR in TTS correlates with the improvement of LV systolic function, confirming the link between microcirculation and myocardial function.[25–28] Coronary microcirculation integrity can also be assessed with myocardial contrast echocardiography (MCE), which helps to detect perfusion defects earlier in LV segments with WMA.[30,31] In addition, MCE enables accurate definition of LV endocardial borders, thus allowing the assessment of LV systolic function and the identification of different morphologic patterns of TTS in patients with poor acoustic windows.[2,32,33]

RISK STRATIFICATION AND FOLLOW-UP

Although TTS patients have generally a favorable long-term prognosis, a variety of complications

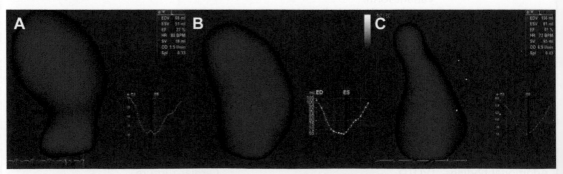

Fig. 3. RT-3DE reconstruction of the left ventricle in 3 patients with TTS during the acute phase. (*A*), the classical apical ballooning with WMA involving the midventricular and apical segments associated with hyperkinesis of the base can be appreciated. The second patient showed at onset a midventricular ballooning pattern, characterized by akinesis of the midventricular segments with relative sparing of the apex and base (*B*). In (*C*), WMAs are confined to the basal segments depicting the morphologic pattern of inverted TTS.

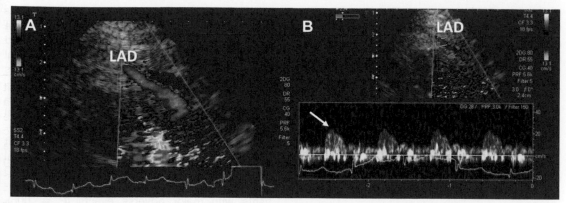

Fig. 4. Adequate flow in the distal tract of the LAD can be clearly visualized despite apical ballooning by transthoracic color Doppler (A). (B) Pulsed-wave Doppler sampling showing a peak diastolic velocity (see *arrow*) of 23 cm/s.

may occur in the early phase.[23,34] In large studies, in-hospital mortality was reported in approximately 2% to 5% of patients with TTS.[8,35] Pulmonary edema is the most common major complication, followed by cardiogenic shock and malignant ventricular arrhythmias.[15] Rarely, LV free wall rupture has been described.[2] TTE is key to detect some mechanical complications, including intraventricular pressure gradients, acute functional mitral regurgitation, right ventricular (RV) involvement, intraventricular thrombi resulting in stroke or arterial embolism, and pericardial effusion. Noteworthy, TTE provides useful parameters for risk stratification.

Left Ventricular Ejection Fraction

LV EF seems to be an independent predictor of major complications, providing additional information for the early identification of patients at higher risk, in particular those aged at least 75 years.[22] EF

less than 40%, together with age greater than 70 years and the presence of physical stressors, are the 3 criteria in the Mayo Clinic score for evaluating the risk of acute heart failure in TTS.[36]

E/e' Ratio

LV diastolic dysfunction, as evidenced by increased E/e' ratio, has been observed in some patients during the early phase of TTS.[3,37,38] Early diastolic untwisting rate, which occurs during LV relaxation, is transiently diminished in TTS,[38] suggesting that at least regional diastolic dysfunction is present (**Fig. 5**). Given that diastolic dysfunction is transient and reversible, the improvement in E/e' ratio at follow-up may be considered as an additional useful indicator of LV function recovery. E/e' ratio is higher in patients with major adverse events and was found to be a significant independent predictor of acute heart failure and in-hospital mortality at multivariate analysis in the Tako-tsubo

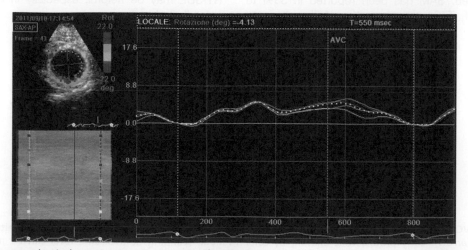

Fig. 5. Decreased apical rotation in a TTS patient. The average peak of apical rotation in this case is of 5°, while in normal subjects it usually ranges from 8° to 12°. This means an impaired twist of the ventricle.

Italian Network (TIN) registry.[15] Keeping in mind that acute heart failure is the most common early complication of TTS, E/e' ratio should be assessed early and systematically to identify patients at higher risk of hemodynamic instability and to guide appropriate management.[2]

Reversible Left Ventricular Outflow Tract Obstruction

LV outflow tract obstruction (LVOTO) may result from basal hypercontractility, as occurs in the typical apical forms of TTS, and may be precipitated or augmented by catecholamine administration.[39] Postmenopausal women with small LV and septal bulge seem to be predisposed to develop this complication.[39] Echocardiographic evidence of significant LVOTO (defined as an intraventricular gradient ≥25 mm Hg, **Fig. 6**) in TTS patients has important therapeutic implications, in particular for patients with advanced systolic heart failure. The prevalence of LVOTO is low, ranging from 12.8% to 25%.[40,41] However, more attention should be paid in such cohorts of TTS patients because of the occurrence of life-threatening arrhythmias and fatal LV wall rupture.[40,41] The degree of reversible LVOTO is variable and depends on loading conditions that should also be monitored by echocardiography. Moreover, it may be associated with systolic anterior motion of the mitral valve (SAM) leading to functional mitral regurgitation.[42,43]

Reversible Mitral Regurgitation

Moderate or severe reversible mitral regurgitation has been demonstrated in about one-fifth of TTS patients (**Fig. 7**).[43–45] The mechanisms underlying mitral regurgitation in TTS are not completely elucidated. SAM has been reported in 33% to 50% of TTS patients with significant mitral regurgitation.[43,44] The occurrence of SAM, especially in case of an intraventricular pressure gradient, further worsens LV pump failure and often induces LVOTO. Significant reversible mitral regurgitation has also been described in patients with severe reduction in LV EF and higher LV volumes in the absence of SAM. These findings suggest that a symmetric tethering of the mitral leaflets secondary to papillary muscle displacement in a dilated and dysfunctional apical left ventricle may have a role in the genesis of mitral regurgitation in this subset of patients.[44] LVOTO and mitral regurgitation are more common in patients with major adverse events (P = .006). Although in a previous small series mitral regurgitation appeared not to significantly influence patient outcome,[45] in the TIN registry, mitral regurgitation has definitely emerged as a powerful prognostic marker associated with cardiogenic shock and in-hospital mortality.[15] Owing to the negative impact on hemodynamic stability and its therapeutic and prognostic implications, LVOTO and significant mitral regurgitation should be ruled out in the early phase of TTS, especially if a new murmur is audible.

Mural or Pedunculated Thrombi

Mural or pedunculated thrombi can be visualized at the apex in 1% to 2% of TTS patients during the first 2 days, causing stroke or systemic embolization (renal or lower limb embolism) in approximately one-third of them.[46] Once thrombus has been documented, therapy with heparin followed by oral anticoagulants should be instituted, and serial TTE should be performed until thrombus resolution and myocardial contractility recovery.[2] In case of diagnostic uncertainty, use of MCE or RT-3DE may be helpful, especially in detecting small thrombi.[2,32]

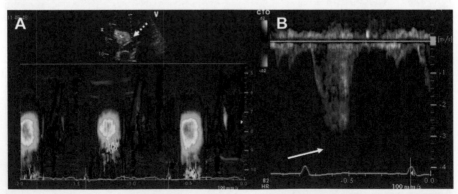

Fig. 6. LVOTO in a TTS patient. (*A*) Interventricular septal bulge predisposing to SAM of the anterior mitral leaflet (*dotted arrow*). Early protosystolic aliasing by color M-mode scanning at the same level can be noted. (*B*) Continuous-wave velocity interrogation of the LVOT in the same patient reveals an intraventricular peak velocity gradient (*solid arrow*) of 36 mm Hg.

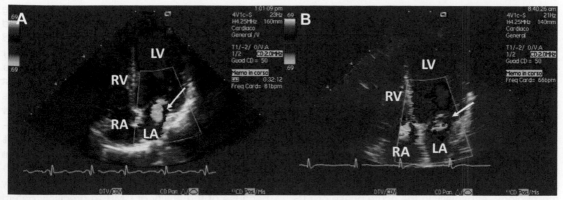

Fig. 7. Reversible MR (*arrows*) in a TTS patient. Moderate mitral regurgitation in the acute phase (*A*) that becomes mild at recovery (*B*) can be appreciated. LA, left atrium; LV, left ventricle; RA, right atrium; RV, right ventricle. (*Adapted from* Citro R, Piscione F, Parodi G, et al. Role of echocardiography in takotsubo cardiomyopathy. Heart Fail Clin 2013;9:6, viii; with permission.)

Right Ventricular Involvement

RV involvement (**Fig. 8**) has previously been associated with a higher incidence of congestive heart failure, cardiopulmonary resuscitation, use of intra-aortic counterpulsation, and longer hospital stay.[47] Owing to its negative impact on patient hemodynamics and cardiac morbidity, special attention should be devoted to detect RV involvement in TTS, particularly in patients with electrocardiographic signs of RV strain pattern. In a large population from the TIN registry, patients with RV involvement experienced acute heart failure in 35.7% versus 13.1% of cases (*P*<.001). Of note, on multivariate analysis, RV involvement had an independent impact on in-hospital outcome.[48]

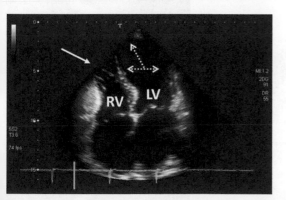

Fig. 8. RV involvement in TTS patients with biventricular ballooning. Apical 4-chamber view: note RV basal hyperkinesis and apex dyskinesis (*solid arrow*), known as inverted McConnell sign. Dotted arrows indicate LV apical ballooning. (*Adapted from* Citro R, Piscione F, Parodi G, et al. Role of echocardiography in takotsubo cardiomyopathy. Heart Fail Clin 2013;9:7, viii; with permission.)

Furthermore 2-dimensional strain may unmask a possible RV involvement. Speckle-tracking echocardiography provides a unique possibility to assess and quantify RV function in the evaluation of patients with TTS, helping the clinician in the differential diagnosis.[49–52]

Pericardial Effusion

Although described with echocardiography only in few cases,[53] using cardiac magnetic resonance (CMR) in 26 TTS patients, Eitel and colleagues[54] reported pericardial effusion in 16 cases (62%). However, because pericardial effusion is not peculiar to TTS and is more commonly associated with an inflammatory process of the myocardium and/or pericardium, it should be always further investigated by CMR in order to rule out myocarditis.

ADVANCED CARDIOVASCULAR IMAGING: CARDIAC MAGNETIC RESONANCE AND CORONARY COMPUTED TOMOGRAPHY ANGIOGRAPHY

Advanced cardiovascular imaging such as CMR and coronary computed tomography angiography (CCTA) in TTS is assuming an emerging role in the diagnosis and management of patients with this syndrome.[54,55] The advantage of both CMR and CCTA is the possibility of evaluating the heart and thorax in multiplanar imaging, overcoming the limits of TTE that are influenced by the acoustic window.[55] Furthermore, compared with coronary angiography (CA) and left ventriculography, these imaging modalities are not invasive.

Not only do CMR and CCTA provide information about LV morphology and function, but they are an adjunctive tool for myocardial tissue characterization and for evaluation of epicardial coronary artery patency, respectively (**Fig. 9**).

Cardiac Magnetic Resonance

The main application of CMR in TTS patients includes the assessment of ventricular morphology and function, and myocardial tissue characterization.

Ventricular morphology and function

Steady-state free precession cine images are required for an accurate assessment of regional and global myocardial function as well as LV morphology, especially in the acute phase of TTS (see **Fig. 9**A).[55]

In a large TTS population of 207 patients examined with CMR within a median of 3 days after presentation, Eitel and colleagues[56] identified 3 main different LV morphologic patterns. The majority of patients (82%) showed the typical apical ballooning with apical akinesia and basal

hyperkinesias, whereas midventricular ballooning and basal ballooning were reported in 17% and 1% of cases, respectively.[56] Furthermore, CMR imaging enables visualization of RV morphology in 3 dimensions and the detection of biventricular involvement. Haghi and colleagues[57] first described RV involvement in 9 of 34 patients (26%) with TTS using CMR performed a few days after TTS onset. Afterwards, Eitel and colleagues[56] observed an even higher rate of 34% of RV involvement in TTS patients. The detection rate of biventricular ballooning in patients undergoing CMR is higher than with TTE, probably because of the ability of CMR to precisely detect even subtle signs of RV involvement that might be missed by TTE. Of note, pleural effusion seems to be more frequent in patients with RV involvement.[57]

Furthermore, delayed enhancement CMR demonstrates higher sensitivity and specificity than echocardiography in detecting LV thrombi,

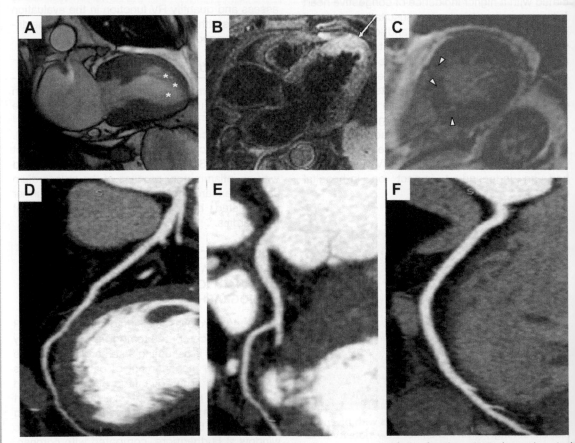

Fig. 9. A 69-year-old patient admitted with suspected ST-elevation myocardial infarction. CMR showed typical apical ballooning caused by hypokinetic midventricular and apical segments (*asterisk, A*). In the same hypokinetic areas, increased signal intensity was evident on T2-weighed sequences (*arrow, B*). Patchy areas of low signal intensity late gadolinium enhancement in the apical septum were detected (*arrowhead, C*). CCTA acquired using a low-dose prospective protocol shows absence of coronary stenosis in the left anterior descending (*D*), circumflex (*E*), and right coronary arteries (*F*).

differentiating thrombi from surrounding myocardium, as thrombus is avascular and does not uptake contrast.[58]

As stated previously, although frequently described also in TTS patients, pericardial effusion is suggestive of an inflammatory status and its detection always requires the ruling out of acute myocarditis using CMR.[54] **Table 2** reports the most common CMR findings in TTS compared with acute myocarditis.

Myocardial tissue characterization

Although the pathophysiological mechanism leading to the development of myocardial edema is still debated (eg, inflammation, transient cardiac ischemia), it represents a typical CMR finding of TTS.[54,59,60]

Owing to the linear correlation of T2 relaxation time with tissue free water, T2-weighted sequences are used to show the presence and extent of myocardial edema (see **Fig. 9**B). In T2-weighted images, a ratio of at least 1.9 between the damaged myocardium and skeletal muscle is considered positive, and usually the location of edema matches the region of WMA with a diffuse or transmural distribution.[56] Thavendiranathan and colleagues[61] used T2 mapping to assess edema in a mixed population of patients with acute myocarditis and TTS in the acute phase. They found that a cut-off value of 59 ms allowed them to identify the area of myocardial involvement with a sensitivity and specificity of 94% and 97%, respectively. Ferreira and colleagues[62] demonstrated that native T1 values are also increased in patients with TTS. These authors found a statistically significant positive correlation between T1 values and T2-weighted ratio (damaged myocardium/skeletal muscle) and a negative correlation between mean myocardial T1 values and systolic dysfunction.[62] In addition, a cut-off value of 990 ms using Shortened Modified Look–Locker Inversion Recovery (ShMOLLI) provided a sensitivity and specificity of 92% for the depiction of the edematous myocardial region.[62] However, the cut-off value of native T1 needs to be evaluated carefully, considering the high variability of normal range using scanners of different fields, vendors, and acquisition schemes.

Of note, in contrast to AMI and myocarditis, in which edema can be visualized for a longer time

Table 2
Main cardiac magnetic resonance findings in patients with Takotsubo syndrome versus acute myocarditis at presentation

	TTS	Acute Myocarditis
LV systolic function	Marked reduction in LV EF on admission with complete recovery at short term	High variability of LV EF. Possible recovery in the form presenting with substantial myocardial dysfunction
Wall motion abnormalities	Circumferential pattern Apical ballooning Variant form: Midventricular ballooning Inverted TTS Biventricular ballooning	Localized or diffuse wall motion abnormalities of the left ventricle and/or right ventricle
Wall thickness	Normal wall thickness	Increased wall thickness
Myocardial edema	High T2 signal intensity with transmural and concentric distribution at sites of wall motion abnormalities	High T2 signal intensity with subendocardial or transmural distribution at sites of wall motion abnormalities
LGE	Usually absent acutely If present acutely, patchy LGE with a focal noncoronary artery distribution, which usually resolves at follow-up	Midmyocardial or subepicardial distribution with a focal noncoronary artery distribution
Additional findings and complications	LVOTO Reversible mitral regurgitation Apical thrombi Pericardial effusion (rare)	Pericardial effusion

Adapted from Lyon AR, Bossone E, Schneider B, et al. Current state of knowledge on Takotsubo syndrome: a position statement from the Taskforce on Takotsubo Syndrome of the Heart Failure Association of the European Society of Cardiology. Eur J Heart Fail 2016;18:7; with permission.

period, in TTS patients, the signal decreases within a few weeks, and so it might not be appreciated at short-term follow-up.[55]

Although many studies pointed out the absence of late gadolinium enhancement (LGE) in TTS, defining it as a criterion for differentiating TTS from other diseases such as AMI and myocarditis, the presence and significance of this finding in TTS have been widely debated.[56,63] Many authors reported LGE in TTS patients, with a prevalence ranging from 9% to 40% (see **Fig. 9**C).[56,64–66] The presence of LGE in TTS was found to depend strictly on the threshold used to identify the areas of hyperenhancement,[56] with no evidence of LGE when a threshold in signal intensity of 5 standard deviations (SD) from remote normally contracting myocardium was used.[66] The lack of LGE when a threshold of 5 SD is applied should be considered in the differential diagnosis with other diseases in doubtful TTS cases.[56] However, the presence of LGE at a lower threshold during the acute phase has prognostic implications, since cardiogenic shock is more prevalent in this subgroup of patients.[66] LGE also disappears at long-term follow-up, but many weeks after edema.[55] Therefore, owing to the peculiar myocardial tissue characterization pattern of TTS, CMR can be used, not only in the acute phase but also during the follow-up in TTS patients who do not show spontaneous WMA recovery in order to consider an ex post alternative diagnosis (**Fig. 10**).[2] Rolf and colleagues[65] demonstrated that the presence of LGE in TTS patients is more dependent on the increase in extracellular matrix, in particular in collagen 1 component, rather than on myocyte necrosis.

The area of LGE in the acute and subacute stage matches with the area of WMA but is not correlated with long-term LV dyfunction.[56,66] Furthermore, normalization of electrocardiographic changes takes longer in patients who test positive for LGE in the subacute stage.[66]

Coronary Computed Tomography Angiography

Although computed tomography (CT) is not considered the technique of choice in patients with TTS, mainly for the exposure to high doses of ionizing radiation, its application in this setting has been described in several cases.[67–69] CT allows for the assessment of cardiac systolic function and the detection of LV WMA, and it might be considered in patients with bad acoustic windows and contraindications for CMR.[70–73] Substantially, CT findings are similar to those provided by CMR, but no information about

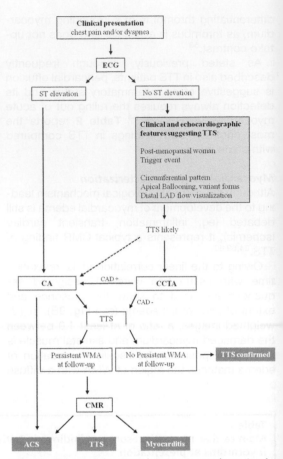

Fig. 10. Proposal for TTS diagnostic work-up in the acute phase and during the follow-up. In patients presenting with chest pain and/or dyspnea and ST-segment elevation, CA should be performed without delay in order to demonstrate culprit coronary lesions or absence of critical stenosis (in the last case ventriculography is recommended). Conversely, in selected patients with clinical and echocardiographic features associated with TTS and no ST-segment elevation on the ECG, CA can be performed within 24 to 48 hours of symptom onset. In this case, CCTA can be performed in order to reduce diagnostic delay. Once critical coronary stenosis has been excluded, echocardiography allows one to monitor WMA recovery. In the case of persistent WMA, CMR should be performed to definitively exclude ACS or myocarditis. ACS, acute coronary syndrome; CA, coronary angiography; CAD, coronary artery disease; CCTA, cardiac computed tomography angiography; CMR, cardiac magnetic resonance; TTS, Takotsubo syndrome; WMA, wall motion abnormalities. (Adapted from Citro R, Lyon AR, Meimoun P, et al. Standard and advanced echocardiography in takotsubo (stress) cardiomyopathy: clinical and prognostic implications. J Am Soc Echocardiogr 2015;28:69; with permission.)

myocardial tissue characterization can be obtained.

The main application of CCTA in TTS patients is in evaluating epicardial coronary arteries to rule out high-grade stenosis (see **Fig. 9**D–F).[33] It is also useful for excluding pulmonary embolism and aortic dissection in patients with acute chest pain and doubtful TTS diagnosis.[2,33] Citro and colleagues[2] proposed CCTA as a noninvasive imaging modality alternative to CA to exclude coronary culprit lesions in patients with no ST-segment elevation at onset and a convincing clinical (postmenopausal woman, trigger event) and echocardiographic (apical ballooning, circumferential pattern, distal LAD flow visualization) picture of TTS to avoid delay in diagnosis, especially when CA is not readily available (see **Fig. 10**). Recently, this approach has been recommended in stable and pain-free patients showing the typical features of TTS, particularly in case of delayed presentation (>48 hours).[35]

MOLECULAR IMAGING

Molecular imaging emerged in the last decade as a possibility of obtaining in vivo images of either functional or molecular processes. Nuclear medicine plays a key role in molecular imaging, since radiotracers allow visualization of cellular function and metabolism, as well as tissue flow without perturbing them. Both single photon emission computed tomography (SPECT) and positron emission tomography (PET) have been applied in TTS using different radiotracers to study innervations, flow, and metabolism.

^{123}I-meta-iodobenzylguanidine (MIBG) is a norepinephrine analog showing the same presynaptic uptake, storage, and release mechanism. ^{123}I-MIBG imaging, both planar and SPECT, is an important tool to evaluate sympathetic function, showing a relevant clinical value for prognostic assessment in several cardiac diseases with a major emphasis in heart failure patients.[74] ^{123}I-MIBG cardiac imaging is performed at 15 minutes (early image) and 3 to 4 hours (late image) after radiotracer administration (111–370 MBq). Although there are some medications (eg, sympathomimetics, combined α/β-blocker, $\beta2$ stimulants, tricyclic antidepressants) and substances (eg, food containing vanillin and catecholamine-like compounds such as chocolate and blue cheese) that may interfere with the uptake of ^{123}I-MIBG, it is possible to perform cardiac imaging in patients on optimal medical therapy.[75] Planar ^{123}I-MIBG cardiac images are analyzed by computing the heart-to-mediastinal (H/M) ratio on both early and late images, as well as the washout rate

(WO) of the tracer from the myocardium between early and late acquisitions. In addition, regional tracer uptake is qualitatively assessed on SPECT images using a 5-point score (from 0 = normal to 4 = no uptake) in a 17-segment model. A reduced late H/M ratio and an increased WO are associated with a poor prognosis, whereas the role of SPECT analysis is still under investigation.[75]

There is evidence showing that epinephrine is an important factor in the pathophysiology of TTS, and ^{123}I-MIBG cardiac imaging offers the unique possibility of investigating the role of cardiac sympathetic innervation.[76] Several studies evaluated ^{123}I-MIBG cardiac imaging in TTS, and the results obtained are consistent, although a relatively low number of patients was studied in each paper.[77–84] Either in the acute or subacute phase of TTS, reduced myocardial uptake of ^{123}I-MIBG in the apical region on both planar and SPECT images has been shown. Interestingly, at disease onset, a reduced late H/M ratio and an increased WO were found, with an increase in the former and a decrease in the latter at follow-up. However, incomplete uptake normalization of ^{123}I-MIBG after 1-year follow-up has been reported.[85] Three examples of late follow-up (6–12 months after onset) are shown in **Fig. 11**. In a recent paper, the effect of α-lipoic acid (ALA) administration, which is known to improve adrenergic cardiac innervations in diabetic cardiomyopathy, was evaluated in TTS.[86] The 48 patients included in the study were randomly assigned to ALA treatment or placebo. In the subacute phase of the disease (14 days after onset), SPECT showed regional reduction in ^{123}I-MIBG uptake in all patients (apical, anterior, apical–septal, apical–lateral, and inferior segments), whereas at 12 months, a significant increase in tracer uptake was observed in the ALA group.[86]

The review of the literature data suggests that ^{123}I-MIBG cardiac imaging has no clinical role in the diagnosis of TTS, mainly because imaging cannot be performed in the first 1 to 2 days after TTS onset due to logistic considerations (ie, the radiotracer should be provided by a commercial source).[77] On the contrary, new insights on pathophysiology could arise from studies with ^{123}I-MIBG. The results reported so far using ^{123}I-MIBG cardiac imaging suggest that TTS could be caused by neurogenic myocardial stunning. A possible explanation for impaired regional ^{123}I-MIBG uptake has been reported, since the pattern of impaired ^{123}I-MIBG uptake follows the increasing b2AR:b1AR ratio from the base to the apex.[87] The phenomenon of persistent reduced regional ^{123}I-MIBG uptake is still unclear, but it could be related to relatively high levels of

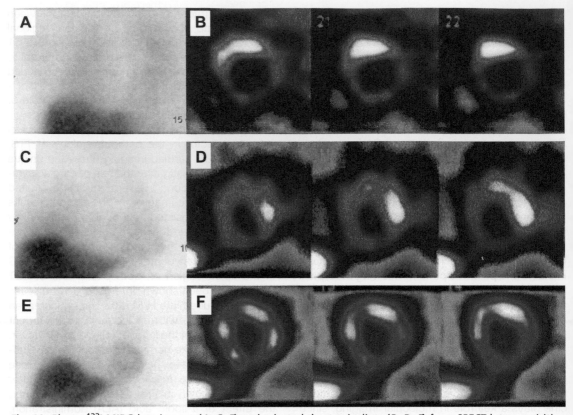

Fig. 11. Planar ^{123}I-MIBG late images (*A, C, E*) and selected short-axis slices (*B, D, F*) from SPECT late acquisition. (*A, B*) Reduced late H/M ratio (1.3) and a clear apical defect on SPECT images. (*C, D*) Mild reduction in H/M ratio (1.5) and a slight apical defect on SPECT images. (*E, F*) Normal H/M ratio (1.8) and normal distribution of the radiotracer on SPECT images.

epinephrine and norepinephrine in the synaptic cleft or to pre-existing myocardial sympathetic denervation. However, since the incidence of sudden death and of disease recurrence is not negligible after discharge in patients with TTS, it could be of interest to evaluate whether the slow recovery of ^{123}I-MIBG uptake may identify those patients who are at an increased risk of recurrence.

PET can be useful for the evaluation of fatty acid metabolism, glucose metabolism, myocardial blood flow (MBF), and innervation. PET scanning has been established for cardiac autonomic innervation assessment, mainly in the research setting. Several radiotracers have been developed and evaluated targeting presynaptic neuronal function, postsynaptic α and β-adrenoceptor density, and second messenger systems. Among them, carbon-11 labeled meta-hydroxyephinephrine ([11C]-mHED), a norepinephrine analog, has been most used. The first large clinical trial (PAREPET [Prediction of Arrhythmic Events with Positron Emission Tomography]) showed that assessment of regional myocardial denervation using [11C]-

mHED predicts sudden cardiac death, independent of EF or infarct volume.[88] In TTS, PET imaging with [11]chydroxyephedrine showed similar findings to those obtained with ^{123}I-MIBG.[89] Until now, ligands for autonomic imaging had only labeled to short half-life radionuclides such as ^{11}C, making it only possible to perform imaging in those centers with an on-site cyclotron. The introduction of ^{18}F labeled tracers for sympathetic innervation will lead to applications in noncyclotron centers, thus allowing for further studies.

The assessment of MBF and CFR with PET might help in understanding TTS. In a pilot study, 3 postmenopausal women underwent adenosine/ rest myocardial perfusion study with nitrogen-13 ammonia and glucose metabolism with ^{18}F-fluorodeoxyglucose PET (FDG-PET) in the acute phase and at follow-up, showing reduced MBF and CFR in the acute phase in the apical versus basal segments, with no change in MBF and improvement in CFR at 3-month follow-up.[90] Furthermore, glucose metabolism was more severely reduced than flow in dysfunctional segments in the acute phase, with an improvement at follow-up.[90] In a study of 25 patients, Christensen and colleagues[91] found that resting MBF was normal in 8 patients (32%) and impaired in 17 patients (68%). In the latter group, the basal regions showed an increase in resting MBF in the acute phase compared with the 4-month follow-up data, whereas in the apical regions resting MBF was reduced in the acute phase and improved at follow-up. Findings from these studies, besides offering new data potentially leading to a better understanding of the mechanisms of TTS, suggest that MBF could have a different pattern in different patients bearing information on clinical outcome.

During the subacute phase (3–20 days after disease onset) FDG-PET showed reduced glucose metabolism with a progressive improvement at follow-up (1–12 months) in hypocontractile apical or mid segments.[82] Moreover, the extent of the metabolic defect was found to be more severe than perfusion abnormality.[90,92] In a series of 13 patients studied in the acute phase and at 2-month follow-up, the typical reduction in FDG uptake in the apical segments was observed in 77% of cases, while in the remaining 23% the anteroseptal region showed glucose metabolism impairment, with normalization of FDG uptake in 82% of all subjects.[93]

All of these data suggest that sudden emotional or physical stress may cause a catecholamine-induced metabolic disorder in the myocardium, which is probably central to this syndrome, suggesting that abnormalities in cardiac glucose metabolism could be associated with TTS. In a recent study, it has been reported that maximal FDG uptake peaked at age 51 to 60 years in females, with a gradual decrease to a minimum FDG uptake at age greater than 70 years, while the opposite has been observed in males.[94] These findings suggest that female hearts depend more on glucose as an energy substrate as they age, probably because of a metabolic link between estrogen and cardiac glucose utilization in people. The authors hypothesized that this characteristic sex-based difference in cardiac glucose uptake might be related to the female predominance of TTS.[94]

Despite being obtained in relatively small populations, the data provided by PET on blood flow and metabolism are consistent and suggest that the pathophysiology of TTS could be related to more complex and inter-related factors.

SUMMARY

TTS is an acute condition characterized by myocardial dysfunction and secondary heart failure. Multimodality imaging is fundamental for a definitive diagnosis.

TTE is the first-line imaging modality for the evaluation of TTS patients. Owing to the possibility of detecting apical ballooning, circumferential pattern, and a wide extension of myocardial dysfunction disproportionate to electrocardiogram (ECG) abnormalities and troponin elevation, TTE is key to reinforce the suspicion of TTS. Beyond diagnosis, TTE allows for the detection of peculiar complications, including LVOTO, reversible mitral regurgitation, RV involvement, intraventricular mural thrombi, and interventricular septum or myocardial wall rupture, useful for risk stratification and appropriate management of patients with cardiogenic shock and hypotension. CMR can be useful to detect myocardial edema in the territory of WMA typically associated with TTS and can help in the differential diagnosis by ruling out other similar conditions (myocarditis and AMI). In addition, CMR improves the ability to recognize RV involvement and small thrombi. CCTA can be used as an alternative to CA to confirm coronary artery patency. Molecular imaging, especially ^{123}I-MIBG cardiac imaging, is a promising technique for the identification of those patients who are at an increased risk of recurrence.

REFERENCES

1. Citro R, Rigo F, Ciampi Q, et al. Echocardiographic assessment of regional left ventricular wall motion abnormalities in patients with tako-tsubo cardiomyopathy: comparison with anterior myocardial infarction. Eur J Echocardiogr 2011;12:542–9.
2. Citro R, Lyon AR, Meimoun P, et al. Standard and advanced echocardiography in takotsubo (stress) cardiomyopathy: clinical and prognostic implications. J Am Soc Echocardiogr 2015;28:57–74.
3. Citro R, Piscione F, Parodi G, et al. Role of echocardiography in takotsubo cardiomyopathy. Heart Fail Clin 2013;9:157–66, viii.
4. Zito C, Carerj S, Todaro MC, et al. Myocardial deformation and rotational profiles in mitral valve prolapse. Am J Cardiol 2013;112:984–90.
5. Cusmà Piccione M, Zito C, Bagnato G, et al. Role of 2D strain in the early identification of left ventricular dysfunction and in the risk stratification of systemic sclerosis patients. Cardiovasc Ultrasound 2013;11:6.
6. Zito C, Sengupta PP, Di Bella G, et al. Myocardial deformation and rotational mechanics in revascularized single vessel disease patients 2 years after ST-elevation myocardial infarction. J Cardiovasc Med (Hagerstown) 2011;12:635–42.
7. Di Bella G, Minutoli F, Pingitore A, et al. Endocardial and epicardial deformations in cardiac amyloidosis and hypertrophic cardiomyopathy. Circ J 2011;75:1200–8.

8. Sosa S, Banchs J. Early recognition of apical ballooning syndrome by global longitudinal strain using speckle tracking imaging—the evil eye pattern, a case series. Echocardiography 2015;32: 1184–92.

9. Heggemann F, Weiss C, Hamm K, et al. Global and regional myocardial function quantification by two-dimensional strain in Takotsubo cardiomyopathy. Eur J Echocardiogr 2009;10:760–4.

10. Heggemann F, Hamm K, Kaelsch T, et al. Global and regional myocardial function quantification in Takotsubo cardiomyopathy in comparison to acute anterior myocardial infarction using two-dimensional (2D) strain echocardiography. Echocardiography 2011;28:715–9.

11. Mansencal N, Abbou N, Pillière R, et al. Usefulness of two-dimensional speckle tracking echocardiography for assessment of Tako-Tsubo cardiomyopathy. Am J Cardiol 2009;103:1020–4.

12. Bybee KA, Kara T, Prasad A, et al. Systematic review: transient left ventricular apical ballooning: a syndrome that mimics ST-segment elevation myocardial infarction. Ann Intern Med 2004;141: 858–65.

13. Hurst RT, Prasad A, Askew JW 3rd, et al. Takotsubo cardiomyopathy: a unique cardiomyopathy with variable ventricular morphology. JACC Cardiovasc Imaging 2010;3:641–9.

14. Templin C, Ghadri JR, Diekmann J, et al. Clinical features and outcomes of takotsubo (stress) cardiomyopathy. N Engl J Med 2015;373:929–38.

15. Citro R, Rigo F, D'Andrea A, et al. Clinical and echocardiographic correlates of acute heart failure, cardiogenic shock and in-hospital mortality: insights from the "Tako-tsubo Italian Network". JACC Cardiovasc Imaging 2014;7:119–29.

16. Fujikawa M, Iwasaka J, Oishi C, et al. Three-dimensional echocardiographic assessment of left ventricular function in takotsubo cardiomyopathy. Heart Vessels 2008;23:214–6.

17. Grabowski M, Piatkowski R, Scislo P, et al. Real-time three-dimensional echocardiography in transient left apical ballooning syndrome. Int J Cardiol 2008;129: e69–70.

18. Schoof S, Bertram H, Hohmann D, et al. Takotsubo cardiomyopathy in a 2-year-old girl: 3-dimensional visualization of reversible left ventricular dysfunction. J Am Coll Cardiol 2010;55:e5.

19. Breithardt OA, Becker M, Kälsch T, et al. Follow-up in Tako-tsubo cardiomyopathy by real-time three-dimensional echocardiography. Heart 2008;94:210.

20. Kurisu S, Sato H, Kawagoe T, et al. Tako-tsubo-like left ventricular dysfunction with ST segment elevation: a novel cardiac syndrome mimicking acute myocardial infarction. Am Heart J 2002;143:448–55.

21. Prasad A, Lerman A, Rihal CS. Apical ballooning syndrome (Tako-tsubo or stress cardiomyopathy):

a mimic of acute myocardial infarction. Am Heart J 2008;155:408–17.

22. Citro R, Rigo F, Previtali M, et al. Differences in clinical features and in-hospital outcomes of older adults with tako-tsubo cardiomyopathy. J Am Geriatr Soc 2012;60:93–8.

23. Sharkey SW, Windenburg DC, Lesser JR, et al. Natural history and expansive clinical profile of stress (tako-tsubo) cardiomyopathy. J Am Coll Cardiol 2010;55:333–41.

24. Meimoun P, Tribouilloy C. Non-invasive assessment of coronary flow and coronary flow reserve by transthoracic Doppler echocardiography: a magic tool for the real world. Eur J Echocardiogr 2008;9:449–57.

25. Meimoun P, Malaquin D, Sayah S, et al. The coronary flow reserve is transiently impaired in takotsubo cardiomyopathy: a prospective study using serial Doppler transthoracic echocardiography. J Am Soc Echocardiogr 2008;21:72–7.

26. Rigo F, Sicari R, Citro R, et al. Diffuse, marked, reversible impairment in coronary microcirculation in stress cardiomyopathy: a Doppler transthoracic echo study. Ann Med 2009;41:462–70.

27. Meimoun P, Malaquin D, Benali T, et al. Transient impairment of coronary flow reserve in tako-tsubo cardiomyopathy is related to left ventricular systolic parameters. Eur J Echocardiogr 2009;10:265–70.

28. Citro R, Galderisi M, Maione A, et al. Sequential transthoracic ultrasound assessment of coronary flow reserve in a patient with Tako-tsubo syndrome. J Am Soc Echocardiogr 2006;19:1402.e5-8.

29. Kume T, Akasaka T, Kawamoto T, et al. Assessment of coronary microcirculation in patients with takotsubo-like left ventricular dysfunction. Circ J 2005;69:934–9.

30. Abdelmoneim SS, Mankad SV, Bernier M, et al. Microvascular function in Takotsubo cardiomyopathy with contrast echocardiography: prospective evaluation and review of literature. J Am Soc Echocardiogr 2009;22:1249–55.

31. Jain M, Upadaya S, Zarich SW. Serial evaluation of microcirculatory dysfunction in patients with Takotsubo cardiomyopathy by myocardial contrast echocardiography. Clin Cardiol 2013;36:531–4.

32. Citro R, Lyon AR, Silverio A, et al. Bubbles in ballooning: safety and utility. J Am Soc Echocardiogr 2015;28:845.

33. Bossone E, Lyon A, Citro R, et al. Takotsubo cardiomyopathy: an integrated multi-imaging approach. Eur Heart J Cardiovasc Imaging 2014;15:366–77.

34. Parodi G, Bellandi B, Del Pace S, et al. Natural history of Tako-tsubo cardiomyopathy. Chest 2011; 139:887–92.

35. Lyon AR, Bossone E, Schneider B, et al. Current state of knowledge on Takotsubo syndrome: a Position Statement from the Taskforce on Takotsubo Syndrome of the Heart Failure Association of the

European Society of Cardiology. Eur J Heart Fail 2016;18:8–27.

36. Madhavan M, Rihal CS, Lerman A, et al. Acute heart failure in apical ballooning syndrome (TakoTsubo/stress cardiomyopathy): clinical correlates and Mayo Clinic risk score. J Am Coll Cardiol 2011;57: 1400–1.

37. Akashi YJ, Goldstein DS, Barbaro G, et al. Takotsubo cardiomyopathy: a new form of acute, reversible heart failure. Circulation 2008;118: 2754–62.

38. Meimoun P, Passos P, Benali T, et al. Assessment of left ventricular twist mechanics in tako-tsubo cardiomyopathy by two-dimensional speckle-tracking echocardiography. Eur J Echocardiogr 2011;12: 931–9.

39. Chockalingan A, Xie GY, Dellsperger KC. Echocardiography in stress cardiomyopathy and acute LVOT obstruction. Int J Cardiovasc Imaging 2010;26: 527–35.

40. Citro R, Previtali M, Bovelli D, et al. Chronobiological patterns of onset of tako-tsubo cardiomyopathy: a multicenter Italian study. J Am Coll Cardiol 2009; 54:180–1.

41. El Mahmoud R, Mansencal N, Pilliére R, et al. Prevalence and characteristics of left ventricular outflow tract obstruction in tako-tsubo syndrome. Am Heart J 2008;156:543–8.

42. Merli E, Sutcliffe S, Gori M, et al. Tako-tsubo cardiomyopathy: new insights into the possible underlying pathophysiology. Eur J Echocardiogr 2006;7:53–61.

43. Parodi G, Del Pace S, Salvadori C, et al. Left ventricular apical ballooning syndrome as a novel cause of acute mitral regurgitation. J Am Coll Cardiol 2007; 50:647–9.

44. Izumo M, Nalawadi S, Shiota M, et al. Mechanisms of acute mitral regurgitation in patients with takotsubo cardiomyopathy. Circ Cardiovasc Imaging 2011;4:392–8.

45. Haghi D, Rohm S, Suselbeck T, et al. Incidence and clinical significance of mitral regurgitation in takotsubo cardiomyopathy. Clin Res Cardiol 2010;99: 93–8.

46. de Gregorio C, Grimaldi P, Lentini C. Left ventricular thrombus formation and cardioembolic complications in patients with takotsubo-like syndrome: a systematic review. Int J Cardiol 2008;131:18–24.

47. Elesber AA, Prasad A, Bybee KA, et al. Transient cardiac apical ballooning syndrome: prevalence and clinical implications of right ventricular involvement. J Am Coll Cardiol 2006;47:1082–3.

48. Citro R, Bossone E, Parodi G, et al. Independent impact of RV involvement on in-hospital outcome of patients with takotsubo syndrome. JACC Cardiovasc Imaging 2015. [Epub ahead of print].

49. Vizzardi E, Bonadei I, Piovanelli B, et al. Biventricular Tako-Tsubo cardiomyopathy: usefulness of 2D speckle tracking strain echocardiography. J Clin Ultrasound 2014;42:121–4.

50. Citro R, Caso I, Provenza G, et al. Right ventricular involvement and pulmonary hypertension in an elderly woman with tako-tsubo cardiomyopathy. Chest 2010;137:973–5.

51. Liu K, Carhart R. "Reverse McConnell's sign?": a unique right ventricular feature of Takotsubo cardiomyopathy. Am J Cardiol 2013;111:1232–5.

52. Hanna M, Finkelhor RS, Shaw WF, et al. Extent of right and left ventricular focal wall-motion abnormalities in differentiating transient apical ballooning syndrome from apical dysfunction as a result of coronary artery disease. J Am Soc Echocardiogr 2007;20:144–50.

53. Ter Bals E, Odekerken DA, Somsen GA. Takotsubo cardiomyopathy complicated by cardiac tamponade. Neth Heart J 2014;22:246–8.

54. Eitel I, Lücke C, Grothoff M, et al. Inflammation in takotsubo cardiomyopathy: insights from cardiovascular magnetic resonance imaging. Eur Radiol 2010;20:422–31.

55. Athanasiadis A, Schneider B, Sechtem U. Role of cardiovascular magnetic resonance in takotsubo cardiomyopathy. Heart Fail Clin 2013;9:167–76, viii.

56. Eitel I, von Knobelsdorff-Brenkenhoff F, Bernhardt P, et al. Clinical characteristics and cardiovascular magnetic resonance findings in stress (takotsubo) cardiomyopathy. JAMA 2011;306:277–86.

57. Haghi D, Athanasiadis A, Papavassiliu T, et al. Right ventricular involvement in Takotsubo cardiomyopathy. Eur Heart J 2006;27:2433–9.

58. Srichai MB, Junor C, Rodriguez LL, et al. Clinical, imaging, and pathologic characteristics of left ventricular thrombus: a comparison of contrast enhanced magnetic resonance imaging, transthoracic echocardiography and transesophageal echocardiography with surgical or pathological validation. Am Heart J 2006;152:75–84.

59. Abdel-Aty H, Cocker M, Friedrich MG. Myocardial edema is a feature of Tako-Tsubo cardiomyopathy and is related to the severity of systolic dysfunction: insights from T2-weighted cardiovascular magnetic resonance. Int J Cardiol 2009;132:291–3.

60. Eitel I, Behrendt F, Schindler K, et al. Differential diagnosis of suspected apical ballooning syndrome using contrast-enhanced magnetic resonance imaging. Eur Heart J 2008;29:2651–9.

61. Thavendiranathan P, Walls M, Giri S, et al. Improved detection of myocardial involvement in acute inflammatory cardiomyopathies using T2 mapping. Circ Cardiovasc Imaging 2012;5:102–10.

62. Ferreira VM, Piechnik SK, Dall'Armellina E, et al. Non-contrast T1-mapping detects acute myocardial edema with high diagnostic accuracy: a comparison to T2-weighted cardiovascular magnetic resonance. J Cardiovasc Magn Reson 2012;14:42.

63. Mitchell JH, Hadden TB, Wilson JM, et al. Clinical features and usefulness of cardiac magnetic resonance imaging in assessing myocardial viability and prognosis in Takotsubo cardiomyopathy (transient left ventricular apical ballooning syndrome). Am J Cardiol 2007;100:296–301.

64. Nakamori S, Matsuoka K, Onishi K, et al. Prevalence and signal characteristics of late gadolinium enhancement on contrast-enhanced magnetic resonance imaging in patients with takotsubo cardiomyopathy. Circ J 2012;76:914–21.

65. Rolf A, Nef HM, Mollmann H, et al. Immunohistological basis of the late gadolinium enhancement phenomenon in tako-tsubo cardiomyopathy. Eur Heart J 2009;30:1635–42.

66. Naruse Y, Sato A, Kasahara K, et al. The clinical impact of late gadolinium enhancement in Takotsubo cardiomyopathy: serial analysis for cardiovascular magnetic resonance imaging. J Cardiovasc Magn Reson 2011;13:67.

67. Nance JW, Schoepf UJ, Ramos-Duran L. Tako-tsubo cardiomyopathy: findings on cardiac CT and coronary catheterisation. Heart 2010;96:406–7.

68. Hara T, Hayashi T, Izawa I, et al. Noninvasive detection of Takotsubo [corrected] cardiomyopathy using multi-detector row computed tomography. Int Heart J 2007;48:773–8.

69. Otalvaro L, Zambrano JP, Fishman JE. Takotsubo cardiomyopathy: utility of cardiac computed tomography angiography for acute diagnosis. J Thorac Imaging 2011;26:W83–5.

70. De Cecco CN, Meinel FG, Chiaramida SA, et al. Coronary artery computed tomography scanning. Circulation 2014;129:1341–5.

71. Lin FY, Min JK. Assessment of cardiac volumes by multidetector computed tomography. J Cardiovasc Comput Tomogr 2008;2:256–62.

72. Tee M, Noble JA, Bluemke DA. Imaging techniques for cardiac strain and deformation: comparison of echocardiography, cardiac magnetic resonance and cardiac computed tomography. Expert Rev Cardiovasc Ther 2013;11:221–31.

73. Pontone G, Andreini D, Bartorelli AL, et al. Diagnostic accuracy of coronary computed tomography angiography: a comparison between prospective and retrospective electrocardiogram triggering. J Am Coll Cardiol 2009;54:346–55.

74. Jacobson AF, Senior R, Cerqueira MD, et al. Myocardial iodine-123 meta-iodobenzylguanidine imaging and cardiac events in heart failure. Results of the prospective ADMIRE-HF (AdreView Myocardial Imaging for Risk Evaluation in Heart Failure) study. J Am Coll Cardiol 2010;55:2212–21.

75. Pellegrino T, Piscopo V, Petretta M, et al. 123I-Meta-iodobenzylguanidine cardiac innervation imaging: methods and interpretation. Clin Transl Imaging 2015;3:357–63.

76. Paur H, Wright PT, Sikkel MB, et al. High levels of circulating epinephrine trigger apical cardiodepression in a beta2-adrenergic receptor/Gi-dependent manner: a new model of Takotsubo cardiomyopathy. Circulation 2012;126:697–706.

77. Madias JE. Do we need MIBG in the evaluation of patients with suspected Takotsubo syndrome? Diagnostic, prognostic, and pathophysiologic connotations. Int J Cardiol 2016;203:783–4.

78. Verberne HJ, van der Heijden DJ, van Eck-Smit BL, et al. Persisting myocardial sympathetic dysfunction in takotsubo cardiomyopathy. J Nucl Cardiol 2009; 16:321–4.

79. Akashi YJ, Takano M, Miyake F. Scintigraphic imaging in Tako-Tsubo cardiomyopathy. Herz 2010;35: 231–8.

80. Mena LM, Martin F, Melero A, et al. Takotsubo syndrome. Usefulness of nuclear medicine studies. Rev Esp Med Nucl 2011;30:104–6.

81. Akashi YJ, Nakazawa K, Sakakibara M, et al. 123I-MIBG myocardial scintigraphy in patients with "takotsubo" cardiomyopathy. J Nucl Med 2004;45: 1121–7.

82. Cimarelli S, Sauer F, Morel O, et al. Transient left ventricular dysfunction syndrome: patho-physiological bases through nuclear medicine imaging. Int J Cardiol 2010;144:212–8.

83. Ito K, Sugihara H, Kinoshita N, et al. Assessment of Takotsubo cardiomyopathy (transient left ventricular apical ballooning) using 99mTc-tetrofosmin, 123I-BMIPP, 123I-MIBG and 99mTc-PYP myocardial SPECT. Ann Nucl Med 2005;19:435–45.

84. Burgdorf C, von Hof K, Schunkert H, et al. Regional alterations in myocardial sympathetic innervation in patients with transient left-ventricular apical ballooning (Tako-Tsubo cardiomyopathy). J Nucl Cardiol 2008;15:65–72.

85. Owa M, Aizawa K, Urasawa N, et al. Emotional stress-induced 'ampulla cardiomyopathy': discrepancy between the metabolic and sympathetic innervations imaging performed during the recovery course. Jpn Circ J 2001;65:349–52.

86. Marfella R, Barbieri M, Sardu C, et al. Effects of α-lipoic acid therapy on sympathetic heart innervations in patients with previous experience of transient takotsubo cardiomyopathy. J Cardiol 2016;67: 153–61.

87. Verschure DO, Somsen GA, van Eck-Smit BL, et al. Tako-tsubo cardiomyopathy: how to understand possible pathophysiological mechanism and the role of (123)I-MIBG imaging. J Nucl Cardiol 2014; 21:730–8.

88. Fallavollita JA, Heavey BM, Luisi AJ Jr, et al. Regional myocardial sympathetic denervation predicts the risk of sudden cardiac arrest in ischemic cardiomyopathy. J Am Coll Cardiol 2014;63:141–9.

89. Prasad A, Madhavan M, Chareonthaitawee P. Cardiac sympathetic activity in stress-induced (Takotsubo) cardiomyopathy. Nat Rev Cardiol 2009;6: 430–4.

90. Feola M, Chauvie S, Rosso GL, et al. Reversible impairment of coronary flow reserve in takotsubo cardiomyopathy: a myocardial PET study. J Nucl Cardiol 2008;15:811–7.

91. Christensen TE, Ahtarovski KA, Bang LE, et al. Basal hyperaemia is the primary abnormality of perfusion in Takotsubo cardiomyopathy: a quantitative cardiac perfusion positron emission tomography study. Eur Heart J Cardiovasc Imaging 2015;16:1162–9.

92. Yoshida T, Hibino T, Kako N, et al. A pathophysiologic study of tako-tsubo cardiomyopathy with F-18 fluorodeoxyglucose positron emission tomography. Eur Heart J 2007;28:2598–604.

93. Rendl G, Rettenbacher L, Keinrath P, et al. Different pattern of regional metabolic abnormalities in Takotsubo cardiomyopathy as evidenced by F-18 FDG PET-CT. Wien Klin Wochenschr 2010;122:184–5.

94. Kakinuma Y, Okada S, Nogami M, et al. The human female heart incorporates glucose more efficiently than the male heart. Int J Cardiol 2013; 168:2518–21.

Takotsubo Syndrome—Scientific Basis for Current Treatment Strategies

CrossMark

Elmir Omerovic, MD, PhD[a,b,*]

KEYWORDS

- Takotsubo syndrome • Left ventricular assist device • Coronary syndrome • Complications

KEY POINTS

- Takotsubo syndrome (TS) is a common acute heart failure syndrome, now increasingly recognized by the medical community.
- TS is characterized by severe reversible left ventricular (LV) wall motion abnormality in the absence of explanatory coronary lesion.
- Despite an increasing number of patients diagnosed with TS worldwide, there are no randomized clinical trials. The fact that TS in most cases is self-healing and, due to the substantial risk of complications, treatment of these patients is challenging and should be based on the PRIMUM NIL NOCERE (first, do no harm) principle.
- In mild cases, no treatment or a short course of limited anticoagulation therapy may be sufficient. Positive inotropic and vasodilating agents should be avoided.
- In severe cases with refractory cardiogenic shock, early treatment with mechanical support using venoarterial extracorporeal membrane oxygenation or a LV assist device should be considered.

INTRODUCTION

Takotsubo syndrome (TS), also known as stress-induced cardiomyopathy, was first reported in 1991 in Japan.[1] It is more frequent in women than men and is often triggered by emotional stress.[1] The syndrome is characterized by a distinctive type of reversible left ventricular (LV) and/or right ventricular (RV) dysfunction with extensive akinesis typically affecting midventricular and apical segments of the heart.[2,3] Although in the majority of cases the patients recover quickly, some patients experience severe cardiac dysfunction causing fulminant heart failure, cardiogenic shock, heart rupture, and ventricular fibrillation leading to death. The late recognition of TS in contemporary medicine may be partly explained by the fact that the initial clinical course of TS is indistinguishable from that of a myocardial infarction and acute heart failure.

The first case of TS in Sweden was recognized and diagnosed in February 2005 at the authors' clinic at Sahlgrenska University Hospital in Gothenburg (a tertiary health care center serving a population of approximately 1,000,000 people), but in retrospective analysis, the authors have identified some cases as early as 1989. Over the past 10 years, the number of diagnosed cases has increased steadily, and at present, the authors diagnose 3 to 5 new TS cases every month, a rate that has been fairly constant over the last couple of years. Because of increasing awareness about the importance of TS, a national TS registry was established within the Swedish Coronary Angiography and Angioplasty Registry (SCAAR) platform[4]

[a] Department of Molecular and Clinical Medicine, Institute of Medicine, Sahlgrenska Academy, University of Gothenburg, Bruna stråket 16, Gothenburg, Sweden; [b] Department of Cardiology, Sahlgrenska University Hospital, Bruna stråket 16, Gothenburg 413 45, Sweden
* Department of Cardiology, Sahlgrenska University Hospital, Bruna stråket 16, Gothenburg 413 45, Sweden.
E-mail address: elmir@wlab.gu.se

Heart Failure Clin 12 (2016) 577–586
http://dx.doi.org/10.1016/j.hfc.2016.06.008
1551-7136/16/$ – see front matter © 2016 Elsevier Inc. All rights reserved.

heartfailure.theclinics.com

in June 2009. Based on data from SCAAR, the authors estimate that as many as approximately 2000 patients develop TS every year in Sweden. The true incidence of TS is likely much higher if one considers that subclinical and milder forms of TS do not receive medical attention. Therefore, despite its late recognition in Europe and worldwide, TS may be the most common form of cardiomyopathy. This syndrome thus deserves full attention and engagement if knowledge is to be advanced and used to improve health outcomes in TS.

TS is acute medical condition. Compared with other common cardiac emergencies (eg, acute coronary syndrome), there is little evidence on which to base treatment recommendations for TS within the concept of evidence-based medicine. Therefore, the patient's safety and best clinical outcome require teamwork involving physicians and medical personnel trained in subspecialties such as interventional cardiology, heart failure, and intensive care who have a special interest in and knowledge of TS. Despite the increasing number of patients with TS and clinicians' awareness of the syndrome, the European Society of Cardiology (ESC) and American Heart Association/American College of Cardiology (AHA/ACC) did not provide support when it comes to treatment recommendations for a long time. Recently, a position statement document from the taskforce on Takotsubo syndrome of the Heart Failure Association of the ESC has been published.[5] This document provides up-to-date relevant information regarding TS pathophysiology, diagnostics, and treatment recommendations grounded on expert opinion. The discussion in this article is based on authors' personal clinical experience from the care of many Takotsubo patients since 2005, as well as on available experimental and clinical evidence in the literature.

GENERAL CONSIDERATIONS ABOUT TAKOTSUBO SYNDROME IN RELATION TO TREATMENT DECISIONS

The most important criterion for diagnosis of TS is spontaneous restoration of normal cardiac function through the process of self-healing, which usually occurs within days or weeks. Consequently, the key objective of in-hospital treatment should be supportive care to minimize complications during recovery. In mild cases, either no treatment or a short course of limited pharmacologic therapy may be sufficient. In severe cases complicated by progressive cardiocirculatory failure, the patients should be considered for mechanical circulatory support early in the clinical

course as a bridge to recovery. Before providing the specific details of optimal treatment strategies, it may be appropriate to provide a short review of current knowledge relevant to the clinical management of TS. The most characteristic hallmark of the syndrome is a development of reversible LV dysfunction with extensive akinesia typically affecting two-thirds (in some cases three-fourths) of apical segments.[2] This leads to cardiac dysfunction that may progress in predisposed patients (due to the natural course of the syndrome or as a consequence of iatrogenic damage) to fulminant heart failure, cardiogenic shock, and, literally, heart rupture, leading to death. Despite the presence of dramatic contractile dysfunction and clinical symptoms during the acute phase, TS is a transient disorder in the majority of patients. Initially, it was believed that TS is a benign syndrome, but contemporary evidence shows that TS is associated with substantial risk of death. Indeed, this risk is similar to that reported in patients with acute coronary syndromes.[3,4,6] The most feared complications in the acute phase are malignant ventricular arrhythmias, thromboembolic complications (eg, stroke, pulmonary embolism), and worsening heart failure leading to cardiogenic shock, all of which may result in loss of life or permanent handicap. What is known about the disease mechanism based on preclinical and clinical observations,[7–13] is that intensive catecholamine overstimulation of the myocardium may be responsible for the development of myocardial dysfunction. However, the optimal treatment for TS remains unknown, as well as which mechanisms are involved in the development of cardiac dysfunction and which pathways are responsible for effective healing.

NEW CLINICAL OBSERVATIONS IN TAKOTSUBO SYNDROME OF IMPORTANCE FOR TREATMENT DECISIONS

Several new observations about clinical manifestations of TS have emerged that are of general importance. It is not unusual for a TS patient to survive an episode in which myocardial akinesia involves approximately 60 to 80% of the left ventricle. In the setting of acute myocardial infarction, loss of function of that magnitude would most likely result in rapid death.[14] Such a contradictory finding highlights on 1 hand the enigmatic nature of TS and on the other hand the limited understanding of the syndrome and therefore the importance of a cautious approach in the process of clinical decision making. One must ask how can it be that most TS patients are hemodynamically fairly stable at rest despite the presence of such an extensive contractile dysfunction. In order to address this question, the authors hypothesized that TS is a cardiocirculatory syndrome.[15] In other words, it is reasonable to assume that compensatory cardiocirculatory mechanisms are activated to maintain sufficient perfusion of the vital organs in the setting of TS. Indeed, the authors' group has demonstrated that TS is associated with decreased sympathetic tone, decreased peripheral vascular resistance, and preserved cardiac output despite extensive apical akinesia.[4] These findings differ from those observed in acute myocardial infarction and are consistent with the observation of near-normal filling pressures in TS.[16] This is yet another counterintuitive finding when compared with acute heart failure due to extensive ischemic damage. Indeed, if one considers that TS is associated with highly elevated plasma levels of catecholamines, it is reasonable to approach TS as a syndrome in which alterations of cardiac and other organ system's function and structure are present simultaneously. In addition to its unique cardiocirculatory profile, TS may be intimately linked to other organ systems. These details suggest an important knowledge gap in the understanding of cardiovascular physiology in general and of TS in particular. In the authors' opinion, it is the combination of the undeniable knowledge gap, the fact that TS in most cases is self-healing, and the presence of substantial risk of death that calls for respect of the fundamental ethical principle PRIMUM NIL NOCERE (first, do no harm) when considering treatment options in patients with TS. Conceptually, one can think of TS as a pathologic condition in which the therapeutic goal is to counteract pathophysiological processes that give rise to the syndrome's multifaceted clinical manifestations. However, one could also think of TS in a fundamentally different way (**Fig. 1**). One could see TS as a protective cardiocirculatory organ response in the setting of high neurohormonal stress. The goal of such a defense mechanism (eg, inhibition of myocardial contractility in larger part of left ventricle) from the evolutionary point of view could be prevention of sudden death. It is well known that high levels of catecholamines and high activity of sympathetic nervous system in the heart are associated with increased risk of ventricular fibrillation due electrophysiological instability. The authors

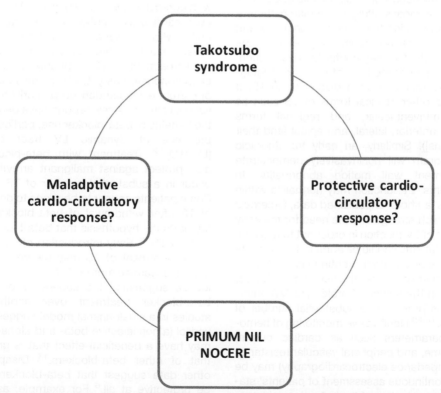

Fig. 1. Conceptual reasoning about TS and consequences for clinical decision making. If TS is a maladaptive response (but self-healing) of which there is limited knowledge, evidence suggests that extrapolation of treatment strategies from acute coronary syndrome and heart failure may be deleterious. On the other hand, TS may be a transient protective cardiocirculatory organ response. In either case, one should apply the central ethical principle PRIMUM NIL NOCERE in clinical decision-making.

proposed this hypothesis previously based on their experimental observations (unpublished data, Redfors B, Shao Y, Omerovic E, 2014) that myocardial infarction in rats (induced experimentally by acute occlusion of left coronary artery) is smaller in animals with experimentally induced TS-like cardiac phenotype (ie, apical akinesia induced by isoprenaline) than in control animals (without TS-like cardiac phenotype). The importance of the PRIMUM NIL NOCERE principle in the care of TS patients becomes even more obvious in the light of possibility that TS may be a protective cardiocirculatory organ response.

INITIAL PATIENT CARE

Once the diagnosis of TS is confirmed, it may be helpful to enquire about previous hospital admissions for chest pain or myocardial infarction. It is not unusual that the index presentation is a recurrence of TS and the previous diagnosis of myocardial infarction was actually TS and not acute coronary syndrome. In the initial phase, standard protocols for management of patients with acute coronary syndrome should be followed until this diagnosis has been convincingly excluded. This is achieved by means of urgent cardiac catheterization demonstrating that coronary anatomy and coronary flow cannot reasonably explain the severity or extent of segmental LV dysfunction. Ventriculography at the time of coronary angiography is essential and often diagnostic in TS. It also reveals other atypical forms of TS such as reversed, midventricular, and regional forms (ie, inferior, anterior, lateral, and apical [and their combinations]). Similarly, an early transthoracic echocardiogram will noninvasively demonstrate and document wall motion abnormality. In some patients, LV function may normalize within 2 to 3 hours (authors' unpublished data, Omerovic E, 2012), which strengthens the need for the early assessment of LV function in order not to miss the diagnosis. Patients should be admitted to an acute cardiac or medical unit with continuous electrocardiogram monitoring, given the risk of arrhythmias, particularly in the setting of prolonged QTc interval, which is present in a substantial number of TS patients.[17–20] Noninvasive monitoring of hemodynamic parameters such as cardiac output, stroke volume, and peripheral vascular resistance (eg, with impedance electrocardiography) may be helpful in continuous assessment of patients' stability and for evaluation of the hemodynamic consequences of pharmacologic treatment. Contrast echocardiography and MRI of the heart in the early phase will exclude LV thrombus and provide further evidence to exclude myocardial infarction.

PHARMACODYNAMIC CONSIDERATIONS IN THE TREATMENT OF TAKOTSUBO SYNDROME

It is important to realize that there are no randomized clinical trials (RCTs) from which one can define the optimal medical treatment and on which one can base recommendations. Consequently, there is large heterogeneity in opinions concerning the best treatment for TS worldwide. Many authors advocate extrapolation of the general knowledge acquired in the field of heart failure, and recommend the use of standard medications such as angiotensin converting enzyme (ACE) inhibitors, beta-blockers, and diuretics. Aspirin (http://www.uptodate.com/contents/aspirin-drug-information?source=see_link) is also suggested for use in the presence of coexisting coronary atherosclerosis. Based on the current evidence implicating catecholamine toxicity in the pathophysiology of TS, the blockade of adrenergic receptors may be a reasonable treatment option. However, whether adrenergic blockade is beneficial, neutral, or deleterious is not known. Some experimental data support the use of beta-blockers in TS.[21] Metoprolol improved the LV ejection fraction in primates with adrenaline-induced TS within 24 hours. However, cardiac dysfunction also normalized in animals who received no treatment. Although several studies were carried out to investigate drug treatment of TS in people, no RCTs have been conducted as yet, which limits the reliability of current evidence derived primarily from observational studies. A few reports have demonstrated the benefits of beta-blocker use, particularly in the presence of dynamic LV tract obstruction (LVOTO).[22] Treatment with beta-blockers may also protect against malignant arrhythmias that occur in a substantial number of TS patients.[23] Some patients appear to be prone to development of TS after withdrawal of beta-blockade, which supports the hypothesis that beta-blockers could prevent TS.[24] Early introduction of beta-blockers in the treatment of TS may theoretically reduce the risk of cardiac rupture.[25] There is no clinical evidence suggesting the superiority of 1 specific beta-blocker treatment over another. Some studies in a small-animal model suggest that carvedilol (a nonselective beta- and alpha-1 blocker) may have a beneficial effect that is greater than that of other beta-blockers.[13] Disappointingly, other data suggest that beta-blockers may not be protective at all.[6] For example, as many as 20% of TS cases occur in patients already receiving beta-blockade treatment.[26] Some small retrospective studies have compared patients treated with traditional cardioprotective medications including beta-blockers, ACE inhibitors, calcium channel blockers, and aspirin with controls.[27,28] There was no difference in LV function at admission and on follow-up, suggesting the ineffectiveness of standard heart failure medications in the prevention and treatment of TS. All this information strengthens application of the do no harm principle. Therefore, in the authors' judgment, for safety reasons, it is prudent not to extrapolate treatment algorithms from heart failure and administer pharmacologic agents such as calcium channel blockers, beta–blockers, and ACE inhibitors to TS patients. One should wait until a better understanding of the pathophysiology behind TS is achieved and until knowledge is acquired from properly designed and conducted RCTs. At the authors' hospital, treatment with beta-blockers and ACE inhibitors is not initiated in the acute phase, respecting the do no harm principle. After normalization (or near-normalization) of segmental function and hemodynamic status, the authors initiate long-term treatment (arbitrarily continued for 1 year) with beta-blockers in the absence of contraindications or intolerance based on the observation that the condition may recur in approximately 15% of patients.[4] In the absence of data from RCTs, the appropriate duration of any therapy for TS is not known.

MILD CASES

Mild cases with rapid symptomatic improvement need no therapy, and early discharge is possible (**Fig. 2**). Some authors advocate conventional heart failure therapy with graded introduction of ACE inhibitors and beta -blockers approved for treatment of heart failure. However, there is evidence that a substantial proportion of TS patients may have altered peripheral sympathetic nerve activity associated with low peripheral vascular resistance.[4] Therefore, administration of ACE inhibitors, beta-blockers, calcium channel blockers or other vasoactive drugs may be harmful. The safety and efficacy of these pharmacologic agents in the treatment of patients with TS have not yet been established.

SEVERE CASES AND CARDIOGENIC SHOCK

A substantial number of patients with TS may present with low blood pressure (BP) but normal or

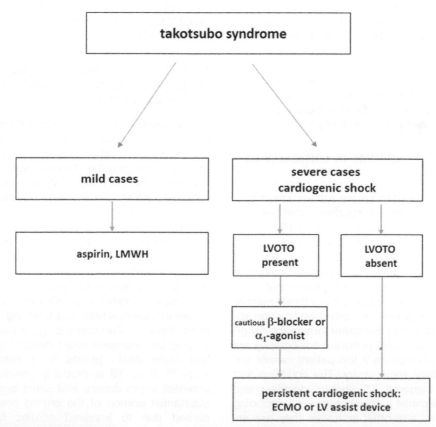

Fig. 2. TS management algorithm.

near normal cardiac output. It is therefore important to provide objective evidence of worsening hemodynamic status (ie, decreasing cardiac output or cardiac index) before making a decision about any pharmacologic treatment that affects (increases or decreases) cardiac contractility and vasomotor activity. TS with severe hemodynamic instability creates unique challenges. The likelihood of acute heart failure and worsening clinical status increases in the presence of higher age (>70 years), presence of a physical stressor, and LV ejection fraction less than 40%.[29] Cardiogenic shock complicating TS is reported in 15% to 20% of patients, pulmonary edema in 20% of patients, ventricular tachycardia in 4% of patients, and death in 5% of patients.[4,26] In TS patients with compromised hemodynamic status, urgent cardiac catheterization with ventriculography or echocardiographic assessment is essential to establish the degree of LV systolic impairment, and to determine the presence or absence of LVOTO. Almost 25% of TS patients develop LVOTO, and treatment of these patients is particularly challenging (see **Fig. 2**).[30] The presence of LVOTO may be recognized already at the time of cardiac catheterization and angiography by after visual inspection of ventriculogram and pull-back across the aortic valve. Some authors recommend cautious treatment with beta-blockers in the presence of dynamic LVOTO based on the rationale that prolongation of diastolic filling time and an increase in LV end-diastolic volume reduces the LVOTO gradient and improves cardiac output.[22,30] Electrical pacing of the RV apex could be considered, if one applies the same reasoning as in the treatment of obstructive cardiomyopathy.

TAKOTSUBO SYNDROME IN CRITICALLY ILL PATIENTS

TS is often triggered by severe somatic stress secondary to life-threatening conditions that one usually sees in the intensive care unit (ICU) such as trauma, bleeding, respiratory insufficiency, infection, or stroke.[5,6] Because it is clinically essential to separate TS from acute coronary syndrome (ACS) as early as possible, it is crucial that coronary angiography is performed in a timely manner in all ICU patients with new-onset wall motion abnormalities. Coronary computer tomography angiography or myocardial perfusion scintigraphy are acceptable alternatives if the patient cannot undergo coronary angiography. The condition that may have triggered TS should identified and treated. Because catecholamines, including noradrenaline, and other inotropes may exacerbate TS, these agents should be contraindicated

in ICU patients in whom clinical course is complicated by TS.[5] There is evidence that catecholamines are associated with a higher mortality in ICU patients with heart failure due to other causes besides TS.[31,32] It is important to recognize that many patients with TS have hypotension caused by low peripheral vascular resistance, but they maintain normal cardiac output. Given the available evidence (clinical and experimental) that implicates primarily signaling through the beta–adrenergic receptor system in the heart for the development of extensive akinesia, phenylephrine (alpha-receptor agonist) rather than noradrenaline (alpha- and beta-receptor agonist) could be used in patients with severe hypotension or in the case of LVOTO with worsening hemodynamic stability. The patient's mental state and subjective assessment of well-being is probably more important that some objective indices such as mean arterial pressure and diuresis when it comes to making a decision about initiation of any inotropic and/or vasoactive pharmacologic therapy. Invasive hemodynamic monitoring may be useful for optimization of fluid balance. Sedatives and other vasodilating drugs should be minimized or avoided. Patients who develop life-threatening hemodynamic instability should be considered for mechanical support with left ventricular assist device (LVAD) or extracorporeal membrane oxygenation (ECMO) as a bridge-to-recovery.

TAKOTSUBO SYNDROME AMONG POTENTIAL ORGAN DONORS FOR HEART TRANSPLANTATION

Today, hearts from many potential donors are discarded when current guidelines for heart transplantation are implemented regarding the presence of regional wall motion abnormalities or impaired cardiac function.[33] Previous reports indicate that 25% to 30% of hearts are discarded due to impaired function in the absence of documented myocardial infarction.[34] Increasing evidence show that TS frequently develops in patients with severe somatic disease. Head trauma, intracranial hemorrhage, and stroke are common precipitators of Takotsubo cardiomyopathy. These conditions are also among the most common causes of brain death among heart transplant donors.[35] Furthermore, TS is thought to be caused by excessive catecholamine stimulation, and brain death results in a catecholamine surge.[36] Thus, TS is probably prevalent among potential organ donors and could account for a substantial portion of the organs presently discarded due to impaired cardiac function or regional wall motion defects. Considering the prognostic benefits associated with heart transplantation and the paucity of donor hearts, identification of additional donors would be of great value.[35] To decrease this organ shortage, the authors have proposed an amendment to current recommendations on donor cardiac function based on anecdotal evidence.[37]

CONCOMITANT CORONARY ARTERY DISEASE IN TAKOTSUBO SYNDROME

Many patients with TS have concomitant coronary artery disease of different severity. Patients with concomitant coronary artery disease should be treated according to the current guidelines based on symptoms and prognostic aspects of revascularization therapy. Patients with life-threatening hemodynamic compromise during the course of acute TS resulting in pulmonary edema and cardiogenic shock pose a particular challenge for clinical decision making at the time of diagnostic angiography. Based on anecdotal evidence from their clinic, the authors recommend complete revascularization when TS is associated with life-threatening hemodynamic instability in the presence of severe coronary artery disease with critical stenosis producing large area at risk (eg, severe stenosis in left main, severe multivessel disease).

POSITIVE INOTROPIC AGENTS

The decision to use sympathomimetic drugs for positive inotropy is challenging and counterintuitive in TS. Given what is known about the mechanisms involved in TS, further activation of catecholamine receptors or their downstream molecular pathways might worsen patients' clinical status and prognosis. Therefore, the use of inotropes such as dobutamine, noradrenaline, dopamine, adrenaline, milrinone, and isoprenaline should be generally regarded as contraindicated in TS. There is solid evidence that catecholamines can directly induce TS,[12] worsen LVOTO by further increasing hypercontractility of the midventricular segment,[38] and delay spontaneous recovery in people. Similarly, administration of adrenaline and isoprenaline induces a TS-like condition in rats[7,13] and mice.[8] The use of the novel inotrope levosimendan in conjunction with noradrenaline has previously been described in patients[39] and in an experimental rat model.[13] The mode of action of levosimendan is different to that of standard inotropes in that it does not act on adrenergic receptors, but rather exerts its positive inotropic effects by prolonging the interaction between actin and myosin. However, this suggestion should be taken

cautiously, as it has been shown in experimental models that levosimendan has adrenergic-like activity, since it inhibits phosphodiesterase[40] and therefore leads to increased levels of intracellular cyclic adenosine monophosphate (cAMP). Furthermore, levosimendan has a pronounced dose-dependent vasodilatory effect, which may further compromise haemodynamic status in an unstable TS patient with low peripheral vascular resistance (PVR). Similarly, in cases where the low cardiac output is associated with low PVR, afterload reduction with intravenous nitrates and ACE inhibitors can be detrimental and should not be used.

MECHANICAL SUPPORT

Intra-aortic balloon counterpulsation (IABP) is recommended by some authors for use in cardiogenic shock caused by TS. IABP improves cardiac output, largely through afterload reduction, and this nonpharmacological therapy has been in use in the treatment of cardiogenic shock for several decades. However, in light of recent neutral data from the IABP-SHOCK II trial[41] and the fact that IABP may worsen dynamic LVOTO, the authors advise against IABP in unstable TS patients. Instead, they advise that patients presenting with worsening hemodynamics and rapid progression to cardiogenic shock and deteriorating multiorgan failure should be considered for early referral for venoarterial ECMO or implantation of LV or biventricular assist device as a bridge to recovery, given that the ventricular function of these patients has an excellent chance of full recovery.[42–44]

PREVENTION OF THROMBOEMBOLISM

TS may be associated with blood hypercoagulability. Indeed, the authors often encounter thromboembolism in their patients, which might reflect the vasoconstrictor, platelet activation, or prothrombotic effects of high catecholamine levels.[45] In their practice, the authors diagnose thromboembolism in approximately 4% of TS patients,[4] which suggests that the potential risk of intraventricular thrombus formation and systemic embolization should be addressed. In the authors' opinion, administration of low-molecular-weight-heparin (LMWH), aspirin, and/or P2Y$_{12}$ receptor antagonists such as clopidogrel, prasugrel, or ticagrelor should be a part of standard treatment and initiated early. Echocardiography and cardiac MRI will provide important information about the presence of mural thrombus and the extent of wall motion abnormality. However, data to ascertain suitable criteria for use of anticoagulation to prevent thromboembolism in patients with TS are scarce. Indirect evidence from randomized trials of anticoagulation for the prevention of LV thrombus formation in large myocardial infarction has shown that the use of anticoagulation for 10 days reduces the incidence of LV thrombus formation. The use of anticoagulation therapy in patients with known LV thrombus is supported by observational studies in which this therapy administered over a period of 4 to 6 months was associated with a reduced rate of embolization. The authors recommend approximately 3 months of anticoagulation if intraventricular thrombus is detected. For patients without thrombus but with severe LV dysfunction, the authors suggest anticoagulation until widespread LV akinesia has been substantially improved or for 3 months, whichever is shorter. Because there is a possibility of TS being complicated by cardiac rupture, it is controversial whether anticoagulation treatment would be advisable. However, the reported number of cases complicated by heart rupture is rather low compared with the number of cases showing an LV thrombus.

PREVENTION OF RECURRENCE

There has been no study that demonstrates effective prevention of recurrence in individuals with TS. Intuitively, beta-blockers may provide some protection against future catecholamine surges, but cases have been reported despite taking beta-blockers, and 1 meta-analysis found no impact upon the risk of recurrence of beta-blockers, albeit with a low frequency of recurrence in both arms.[46,47] The role of psychological counseling and cognitive behavioral therapy remains to be determined, but they may have a role in selected cases with recurrence triggered by emotional stressors, and also in cases where anxiety disorder is confirmed.

SUMMARY AND FUTURE DIRECTIONS

TS is a common and fascinating acute heart failure syndrome, now increasingly recognized by the medical community. Many facets of this clinical entity are incompletely understood, which limits the knowledge foundation on which to base recommendations for optimal clinical management. However, the increasing incidence and the high frequency of complications during the acute phase reinforce the need to improve care pathways for individuals with TS.

REFERENCES

1. Nef HM, Mollmann H, Akashi YJ, et al. Mechanisms of stress (Takotsubo) cardiomyopathy. Nat Rev Cardiol 2010;7:187–93.
2. Wittstein IS, Thiemann DR, Lima JA, et al. Neurohumoral features of myocardial stunning due to sudden emotional stress. N Engl J Med 2005;352:539–48.
3. Redfors B, Vedad R, Angerås O, et al. Mortality in takotsubo syndrome is similar to mortality in myocardial infarction—a report from the SWEDEHEART registry. Int J Cardiol 2015;185:282–9.
4. Schultz T, Shao Y, Redfors B, et al. Stress-induced cardiomyopathy in Sweden: evidence for different ethnic predisposition and altered cardio-circulatory status. Cardiology 2012;122:180–6.
5. Lyon AR, Bossone E, Schneider B, et al. Current state of knowledge on Takotsubo syndrome: a position statement from the Taskforce on Takotsubo Syndrome of the Heart Failure Association of the European Society of Cardiology. Eur J Heart Fail 2016;18(1):8–27.
6. Templin C, Ghadri JR, Diekmann J, et al. Clinical features and outcomes of Takotsubo (stress) cardiomyopathy. N Engl J Med 2015;373:929–38.
7. Shao Y, Redfors B, Scharin Tang M, et al. Novel rat model reveals important roles of beta-adrenoreceptors in stress-induced cardiomyopathy. Int J Cardiol 2013;168:1943–50.
8. Shao Y, Redfors B, Stahlman M, et al. A mouse model reveals an important role for catecholamine-induced lipotoxicity in the pathogenesis of stress-induced cardiomyopathy. Eur J Heart Fail 2013;15:9–22.
9. Ellison GM, Torella D, Karakikes I, et al. Acute beta-adrenergic overload produces myocyte damage through calcium leakage from the ryanodine receptor 2 but spares cardiac stem cells. J Biol Chem 2007;282:11397–409.
10. Ueyama T, Ishikura F, Matsuda A, et al. Chronic estrogen supplementation following ovariectomy improves the emotional stress-induced cardiovascular responses by indirect action on the nervous system and by direct action on the heart. Circ J 2007;71:565–73.
11. Ueyama T, Kasamatsu K, Hano T, et al. Catecholamines and estrogen are involved in the pathogenesis of emotional stress-induced acute heart attack. Ann N Y Acad Sci 2008;1148:479–85.
12. Abraham J, Mudd JO, Kapur NK, et al. Stress cardiomyopathy after intravenous administration of catecholamines and beta-receptor agonists. J Am Coll Cardiol 2009;53:1320–5.

13. Paur H, Wright PT, Sikkel MB, et al. High levels of circulating epinephrine trigger apical cardiodepression in a beta2-adrenergic receptor/Gi-dependent manner: a new model of Takotsubo cardiomyopathy. Circulation 2012;126: 697–706.

14. Page DL, Caulfield JB, Kastor JA, et al. Myocardial changes associated with cardiogenic shock. N Engl J Med 1971;285:133–7.

15. Redfors B, Shao Y, Ali A, et al. Are the different patterns of stress-induced (Takotsubo) cardiomyopathy explained by regional mechanical overload and demand: supply mismatch in selected ventricular regions? Med Hypotheses 2013;81: 954–60.

16. Redfors B, Shao Y, Ali A, et al. Rat models reveal differences in cardiocirculatory profile between Takotsubo syndrome and acute myocardial infarction. J Cardiovasc Med (Hagerstown) 2015;16:632–8.

17. Akashi YJ, Nef HM, Mollmann H, et al. Stress cardiomyopathy. Annu Rev Med 2010;61:271–86.

18. Bonello L, Com O, Ait-Moktar O, et al. Ventricular arrhythmias during Takotsubo syndrome. Int J Cardiol 2008;128:e50–3.

19. Mahida S, Dalageorgou C, Behr ER. Long-QT syndrome and torsades de pointes in a patient with Takotsubo cardiomyopathy: an unusual case. Europace 2009;11:376–8.

20. Matsuoka K, Okubo S, Fujii E, et al. Evaluation of the arrhythmogenecity of stress-induced "Takotsubo cardiomyopathy" from the time course of the 12-lead surface electrocardiogram. Am J Cardiol 2003;92:230–3.

21. Izumi Y, Okatani H, Shiota M, et al. Effects of metoprolol on epinephrine-induced takotsubo-like left ventricular dysfunction in non-human primates. Hypertens Res 2009;32:339–46.

22. Migliore F, Bilato C, Isabella G, et al. Haemodynamic effects of acute intravenous metoprolol in apical ballooning syndrome with dynamic left ventricular outflow tract obstruction. Eur J Heart Fail 2010;12: 305–8.

23. Dib C, Prasad A, Friedman PA, et al. Malignant arrhythmia in apical ballooning syndrome: risk factors and outcomes. Indian Pacing Electrophysiol J 2008;8:182–92.

24. Jefic D, Koul D, Boguszewski A, et al. Transient left ventricular apical ballooning syndrome caused by abrupt metoprolol withdrawal. Int J Cardiol 2008; 131:E35–7.

25. Kumar S, Kaushik S, Nautiyal A, et al. Cardiac rupture in takotsubo cardiomyopathy: a systematic review. Clin Cardiol 2011;34:672–6.

26. Sharkey SW, Windenburg DC, Lesser JR, et al. Natural History and Expansive Clinical Profile of Stress (Tako-Tsubo) Cardiomyopathy. J Am Coll Cardiol 2010;55:333–41.

27. Fazio G, Pizzuto C, Barbaro G, et al. Chronic pharmacological treatment in takotsubo cardiomyopathy. Int J Cardiol 2008;127:121–3.

28. Kurisu S, Inoue I, Kawagoe T, et al. Assessment of medications in patients with tako-tsubo cardiomyopathy. Int J Cardiol 2009;134:E120–3.

29. Madhavan M, Rihal CS, Lerman A, et al. Acute heart failure in apical ballooning syndrome (Takotsubo/stress cardiomyopathy): clinical correlates and Mayo Clinic risk score. J Am Coll Cardiol 2011;57: 1400–1.

30. Fefer P, Chelvanathan A, Dick AJ, et al. Takotsubo cardiomyopathy and left ventricular outflow tract obstruction. J Interv Cardiol 2009;22:444–52.

31. Tacon CL, McCaffrey J, Delaney A. Dobutamine for patients with severe heart failure: a systematic review and meta-analysis of randomised controlled trials. Intensive Care Med 2012;38: 359–67.

32. Redfors B, Omerovic E. Takotsubo (stress) cardiomyopathy. N Engl J Med 2015;373:2688–9.

33. Costanzo MR, Dipchand A, Starling R, et al. The International Society of Heart and Lung Transplantation Guidelines for the care of heart transplant recipients. J Heart Lung Transplant 2010; 29:914–56.

34. Boudaa C, Lalot JM, Perrier JF, et al. Evaluation of donor cardiac function for heart transplantation: experience of a French academic hospital. Ann Transplant 2000;5:51–3.

35. Lund LH, Edwards LB, Kucheryavaya AY, et al. The Registry of the International Society for Heart and Lung Transplantation: thirtieth official adult heart transplant report–2013; focus theme: age. J Heart Lung Transplant 2013;32:951–64.

36. Perez Lopez S, Otero Hernandez J, Vazquez Moreno N, et al. Brain death effects on catecholamine levels and subsequent cardiac damage assessed in organ donors. J Heart Lung Transplant 2009;28:815–20.

37. Redfors B, Ramunddal T, Oras J, et al. Successful heart transplantation from a donor with Takotsubo syndrome. Int J Cardiol 2015;195:82–4.

38. Yoshioka T, Hashimoto A, Tsuchihashi K, et al. Clinical implications of midventricular obstruction and intravenous propranolol use in transient left ventricular apical ballooning (Tako-tsubo cardiomyopathy). Am Heart J 2008;155(526): e521–7.

39. Padayachee L. Levosimendan: the inotrope of choice in cardiogenic shock secondary to takotsubo cardiomyopathy? Heart Lung Circ 2007;16(Suppl 3): S65–70.

40. Ajiro Y, Hagiwara N, Katsube Y, et al. Levosimendan increases L-type Ca(2+) current via phosphodiesterase-3 inhibition in human cardiac myocytes. Eur J Pharmacol 2002;435:27–33.

41. Thiele H, Zeymer U, Neumann FJ, et al. Intraaortic balloon support for myocardial infarction with cardiogenic shock. N Engl J Med 2012;367:1287–96.

42. Bonacchi M, Valente S, Harmelin G, et al. Extracorporeal life support as ultimate strategy for refractory severe cardiogenic shock induced by Takotsubo cardiomyopathy: a new effective therapeutic option. Artif Organs 2009;33:866–70.

43. Redfors B, Shao Y, Omerovic E. Stress-induced cardiomyopathy in a patient with chronic spinal cord transection at the level of C5: endocrinologically mediated catecholamine toxicity. Int J Cardiol 2012;159(3):e61–2.

44. Bonacchi M, Maiani M, Harmelin G, et al. Intractable cardiogenic shock in stress cardiomyopathy with left ventricular outflow tract obstruction: is extracorporeal life support the best treatment? Eur J Heart Fail 2009;11:721–7.

45. Akashi YJ, Goldstein DS, Barbaro G, et al. Takotsubo cardiomyopathy: a new form of acute, reversible heart failure. Circulation 2008;118: 2754–62.

46. Santoro F, Ieva R, Musaico F, et al. Lack of efficacy of drug therapy in preventing takotsubo cardiomyopathy recurrence: a meta-analysis. Clin Cardiol 2014;37(7):434–9.

47. Palla AR, Dande AS, Petrini J, et al. Pretreatment with low-dose beta-adrenergic antagonist therapy does not affect severity of Takotsubo cardiomyopathy. Clin Cardiol 2012;35: 478–81.

Takotsubo Syndrome
Insights from Japan

Yoshihiro J. Akashi, MD, PhD, FESC, FJCC[a],*, Masaharu Ishihara, MD, PhD, FACC, FJCC[b]

KEYWORDS

- Apical ballooning • Autonomic nervous • Catecholamine • Estrogen • Stress • Heart failure

KEY POINTS

- *Takotsubo* has been used as a pot/vase for catching octopus in Japan since several centuries BCE; this name was first used as myocardial phenomenon in 1990.
- Emotional and physical stress, such as a big earthquake, can trigger takotsubo syndrome.
- No treatment regimen for patients with takotsubo syndrome has been established because of lack of evidence.
- Prospective clinical trials will be required for hypothesis testing based on animal experiments.

INTRODUCTION

In this quarter of century, a novel cardiac syndrome with transient left ventricular dysfunction has been described all over the world. This entity has been known as takotsubo cardiomyopathy, named for the particular shape of the end-systolic left ventricle on the left ventriculograms. Currently, some Japanese clinicians acknowledge that this type of reversible heart failure existed before the actual name was defined. Japanese name *takotsubo* draws attention in the field of heart failure. In this article, as representatives of the country of name origin, we report the history and new insights of takotsubo syndrome based on the achievements that many Japanese researchers contributed to benefit in the field of cardiology.

HISTORY

Takotsubo syndrome is situated as a primary acquired cardiomyopathy according to the American Heart Association classification,[1] although it has been recently considered as a different entity from cardiomyopathy.[2] This syndrome includes tako-tsubo cardiomyopathy,[3] stress cardiomyopathy,[4] apical ballooning,[5] and "broken heart."[6] A takotsubo is a Japanese octopus trap widely used around Akashi Channel in Hyogo prefecture and Seto Inland Sea from several centuries BCE (**Fig. 1**). In 1990, the term *takotsubo* was first described in the medical literature by Dr Hikaru Sato,[7] from Hiroshima City Hospital in Hiroshima, Japan. The title of this report was "tsubo-shaped" stunned myocardium written in Japanese, English title was renamed as "tako-tsubo–like left ventricular dysfunction."[7] *Tsubo-shaped* means *potlike*. In 1991, Dr Dote,[8] one of Dr Sato's colleagues, presented a study entitled "Myocardial stunning due to simultaneous multivessel coronary spasm," which was the first takotsubo case series published in a peer-reviewed journal in Japanese with an English abstract. This study report was cited frequently by numerous scientific journals because of the impressive figures, including 5 cases depicted by using left ventriculography. According to the Scopus search engine, it was

Conflicts of Interest: None.
Disclosure: Nothing.
[a] Division of Cardiology, Department of Internal Medicine, St. Marianna University School of Medicine, 2-16-1 Sugao Miyamae-ku, Kawasaki, Kanagawa, 216-8511, Japan; [b] Division of Coronary Artery Disease, Department of Internal Medicine, Hyogo College of Medicine, 1-1, Mukogawa-cho, Nishinomiya, Hyogo 663-8501, Japan
* Corresponding author.
E-mail address: yoakashi-circ@umin.ac.jp

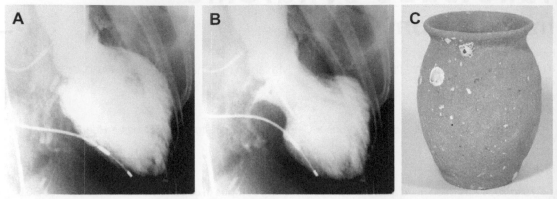

Fig. 1. Left ventriculograms in the right anterior oblique projection. (*A*) In the end-diastolic phase. (*B*) In the end-systolic phase. The extensive area around the apex shows akinesis; the basal segments display hypercontraction, particularly in the end-diastolic phase. (*C*) A picture of a real *takotsubo*. (*Adapted from* Akashi YJ, Goldstein DS, Barbaro G, et al. Takotsubo cardiomyopathy: a new form of acute, reversible heart failure. Circulation 2008;118:2755; with permission.)

quoted for the scientific journal more than 700 times. In the abstract, takotsubo was first expressed with Chinese characters.

In 1986, the *New England Journal of Medicine* presented a case of 44-year-old female complaining her chest pain after severe emotional stress.[9] It is presumed to be the first reported case of takotsubo syndrome outside Japan; however, the name of takotsubo or takotsubo phenomenon was not known at that time. In 1977, Dr Kuramoto reported 7 cases of acute reversible myocardial infarction after blood transfusion in elderly patients.[10] Although his study presented no findings of left ventriculograms or echocardiograms, the time course recorded by electrocardiography was quite similar to that in patients with takotsubo syndrome.

EARTHQUAKE

Japan often suffers earthquakes and the oldest earthquake was recorded in the seventh century CE. In the last few decades, 3 great earthquakes have struck Japan. In the Great Hanshin-Awaji earthquake in 1995, the prevalence of deep negative T wave on the electrocardiograms was reported frequently.[11] Although the incidence of acute myocardial infarction (AMI) significantly increased after this earthquake,[12] this T-wave inversion might include some patients with AMI. Yamabe and colleagues[11] presented the defect in the left ventricular apex on ^{123}I-metaiodobenzylguanidine (^{123}I-MIBG) myocardial scintigraphic images within several months after the earthquake, whereas myocardial perfusion single photon emission computed tomography imaging revealed no defects in the left ventricle. Looking back of these

phenomena, those cases should have been included as takotsubo syndrome.

Takotsubo syndrome became the focus of attention after the Niigata Chuetsu earthquake in 2004 in Japan.[13] The number of patients who presented with takotsubo syndrome within 1 week after the Niigata Chuetsu earthquake was equivalent to that of those for the previous 10 years. One study reported as follows: (1) the prevalence of takotsubo syndrome after the Great East Japan earthquake in 2011 was lower than that of the Niigata Chuetsu earthquake and (2) the number of patients suffering from this syndrome was lower than expected.[14] Meanwhile, a certain number of patients with this syndrome was reported after the earthquakes in Christchurch, New Zealand, in 2010 and in 2011.[15] The onset of takotsubo syndrome is definitely associated with the disaster, such as earthquakes.

EVIDENCE FROM JAPAN

A large number of evidence concerning takotsubo syndrome has been presented from Japan as follows.

Nuclear Imaging

Several study papers using the imaging modalities in patients with takotsubo syndrome have been published in Japan. Ito and colleagues[16] demonstrated first nuclear study in 2001. They administrated thechnetium-99m-tetrofosmin and ^{123}I-β-methyl-iodophenyl pentadecanoic acid (^{123}I-BMIPP) to patients without coronary disease who revealed stunned myocardium after contrast medium administration. They focused on the administration of ^{123}I-BMIPP and the total defect scores (TDS) of thechnetium-99m-tetrofosmin in the acute, subacute, and chronic phases (1 month after onset) in those patients. The TDS was the highest in the acute phase compared with the subacute and chronic phases. Thallium-201 myocardial scintigraphy was also studied by Kurisu and colleagues[17]; the TDS of thallium-201 was lower than that of ^{123}I-BMIPP in the acute phase. The most recent study conducted by Matsuo and colleagues[18] has proposed that the TDS of ^{123}I-BMIPP in patients with takotsubo syndrome is trivial than that of in those with AMI.

The findings from ^{123}I-MIBG myocardial scintigraphic imaging are also presented. In 2001, Owa and colleagues[19] reported that the recovery of ^{123}I-MIBG uptake was slower than that of the other tracers. ^{123}I-MIBG imaging combined with myocardial perfusion scintigraphy depicts abnormal myocardial sympathetic innervation in a pattern consistent with one of the variants of takotsubo syndrome in the absence of a myocardial perfusion abnormality or scar.[20,21] ^{123}I-MIBG imaging also has a possibility to prevent excessive adrenal and ectopic catecholamine secretion while using whole body imaging with the same tracer, such as pheochromocytoma.[22] Because ^{123}I-MIBG myocardial scintigraphic imaging is quite useful to follow cardiac sympathetic activities in patients with takotsubo syndrome, the Task Force on Takotsubo Syndrome of the Heart Failure Association of the European Society of Cardiology insists in their position statement that the recovery of ventricular systolic dysfunction on cardiac images at follow-up is required for accurate diagnosis of this syndrome.[2] The authors previously conducted a study to prove autonomic dysfunction in patients with takotsubo syndrome and analyzed heart rate variability using Holter monitoring.[23]

The first clinical study with PET in Japan by Yoshida and colleagues[24] demonstrated remarkably reduced uptake of ^{18}F FDG PET in the apex despite slightly reduced uptake of perfusion tracer. No PET study from Japan has been reported after the publication of Yoshidas' study, although some of the impressive images were presented in the *European Heart Journal*.[25]

Echocardiography

Echocardiography is a promising modality to detect the wall motion abnormalities simply and easily in the clinical setting, although only a handful of clinical studies using echocardiography have been published in Japan. One of the mechanisms of acute mitral regurgitation in patients with takotsubo syndrome was clarified because many patients complicated with acute heart failure owing to mitral regurgitation in their acute phase of takotsubo syndrome.[26] The changes in the mitral valve observed in approximately 25% of patients in their acute phase were improved after the wall motion was normalized. Some researchers focused on the secondary pulmonary hypertension owing to mitral regurgitation in patients with takotsubo syndrome.[27] Effective regurgitant orifice area of mitral regurgitation evaluated by 2-dimensioanl Doppler echocardiography was associated with pulmonary artery systolic pressure and the acute phase of the effective regurgitant orifice area was an independent predictor for pulmonary artery systolic pressure in these patients. Greater pulmonary artery systolic pressure was associated with the signs of shortness of breath.

Electrocardiography

ST-segment elevation and/or T-wave inversion is always observed in patients with takotsubo syndrome. The prevalence of these changes depends on the time from the onset of this syndrome. It is usually difficult to distinguish the patients with takotsubo syndrome from those with acute anterior AMI based on electrocardiographic findings; however, Japanese researchers attempted to prove the usefulness of electrocardiography to differentiate takotsubo syndrome from AMI. Kosuge and colleagues[28] first demonstrated the difference of electrocardiographic findings between takotsubo syndrome and AMI in Japan. Patients with anterior AMI have ST-segment elevation in leads V_2 to V_4. Meanwhile, ST-segment elevation most frequently occurred in lead −aVR facing the apical and inferolateral regions in patients with takotsubo syndrome. V_1 in takotsubo syndrome is the wall motion abnormalities in takotsubo syndrome less frequently extending to the V_1-lead region (**Fig. 2**). Owing to these findings, cardiologists are able to differentiate classical apical type of takotsubo syndrome from anterior AMI with the sensitivity and specificity of 90% or more.[28] Kosuge and colleagues[29] also investigated T-wave inversion and reported that negative T waves in lead −aVR (ie, positive T waves in lead aVR) and no negative T waves in lead V_1 were identified in takotsubo syndrome with a sensitivity of 95% and a specificity of 97% (**Fig. 3**). When the left anterior descending coronary artery is wrapped into the left ventricular apex, it is difficult to distinguish a typical case with takotsubo syndrome from anterior AMI whose culprit lesion is distal to left anterior descending coronary artery.

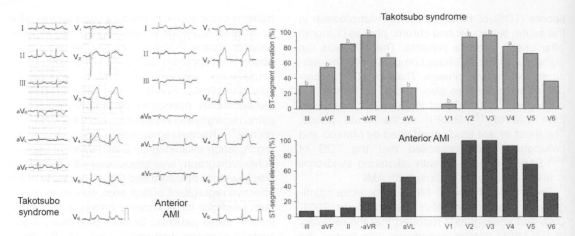

Fig. 2. Representative electrocardiograms (*left*) and prevalence of ST-segment elevation (*right*). Takotsubo syndrome is more frequently associated with ST-segment elevation in leads III, aVF, II, aVR, and I, particularly in lead aVR, and less frequently associated with ST-segment elevation in leads aVL and V_1 to V_4, particularly in lead V_1 ([a] $P < .05$, [b] $P < .01$ vs anterior acute myocardial infarction [AMI]). (*Adapted from* Kosuge M, Ebina T, Hibi K, et al. Simple and accurate electrocardiographic criteria to differentiate takotsubo cardiomyopathy from anterior acute myocardial infarction. J Am Coll Cardiol 2010;55:2515; with permission.)

Shimizu and colleagues[30] investigated the significance of presence of J-wave in patients with takotsubo syndrome. In their analysis, the existence of J-wave was greater in the lethal group after cardiac death and/or ventricular tachyarrhythmia; thus, J-wave was the best predictor for lethality in the multivariate stepwise logistic regression analysis.[30]

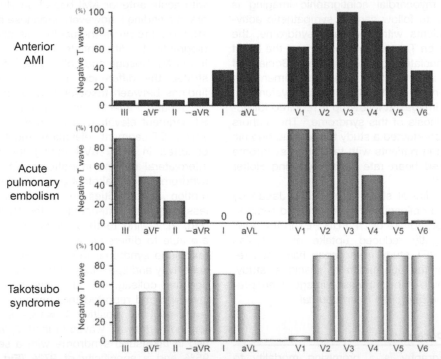

Fig. 3. Prevalence of negative T waves in patients with acute coronary syndrome, acute pulmonary embolism (APE) and takotsubo syndrome. According to their results, negative T waves in both leads III and V_1 identified APE with a sensitivity of 90% and a specificity of 97%. Negative T waves in lead –aVR (ie, positive T waves in lead aVR) and no negative T waves in lead V_1 identified takotsubo syndrome (with a sensitivity of 95% and a specificity of 97%). (*Adapted from* Kosuge M, Ebina T, Hibi K, et al. Differences in negative T waves among acute coronary syndrome, acute pulmonary embolism, and takotsubo cardiomyopathy. European Heart Journal Acute Cardiovascular Care 2012;1:352; with permission.)

From Registry Database

In Japan, several registry data regarding takotsubo syndrome has been published. The member of Angina Pectoris-Myocardial Infarction (AP-MI) investigators approved one 1 dataset obtained from 88 patients with takotsubo syndrome collected between 1991 and 2000.[31] This was the first registry data for takotsubo syndrome in the world. They demonstrated the precise clinical features of this syndrome. Of the study patients, 90% patients revealed ST elevation on the electrocardiograms and 97% patients had T wave inversion; of note, 2.7% patients had a recurrent episode.[31]

Another dataset was approved by the Tokyo CCU Network, a working group for takotsubo syndrome. They documented the incidence of complications and seasonal distribution of the disease onset during 1 year in 107 recorded patients.[32] As **Fig. 4** shows, the twin peaks were observed and the change of seasons seemed to trigger this syndrome. Of these, 37 patients experienced complications, such as pump failure and 67 patients had no complications. In their analysis, the initial concentration of plasma brain natriuretic peptide was the best predictor for in-hospital cardiac complications (odds ratio, 4.92; 95% CI, 1.97–12.3; $P = .001$).[32] Murakami and colleagues[33] recently presented the other analytics results from the same registry data; of the 368 recorded patients, women tended to suffer from takotsubo syndrome and male patients with this syndrome had more cardiac events than female patients (**Fig. 5**).[33]

The other data were from the Broad-range Organization for Renal, Arterial and cardiac studies (BOREAS) conducted by Sapporo Medical University Affiliates Registry.[34] Data from 251 patients were used to identify the survival difference between the takotsubo patients with the classical contractile pattern and those with the variant contractile type. No differences in prognosis were found between the 2 groups. Midventricular obstruction would be the determinant of recurrence (odds ratio, 14.71; 95% CI, 1.87–304.66; $P = .01$); meanwhile, older age (odds ratio, 1.09; 95% CI, 1.02–1.17; $P < .01$) and cardiogenic shock could be the risk factor for cardiac death (odds ratio, 4.27; 95% CI, 1.07–18.93; $P = .04$). Moreover, the other group in Japan analyzed this data and they demonstrated that left ventricular outflow obstruction was associated with the recurrence of takotsubo syndrome.[35]

Diagnosis Procedure Combination

From 2002, Japan has introduced the diagnosis procedure combination as a patient classification system for the medical institutions, which was launched by the Ministry of Health, Labor and Welfare of Japan. This is quite similar to the diagnosis-related groups used for Medicare in the United States. The diagnosis procedure combination evaluates the quality and cost of medical services in Japan. From this database, Isogai and colleagues[36] assessed the difference in pathogenesis in inpatients and outpatients with takotsubo syndrome. This largest existing data in Japan provided useful information on the takotsubo syndrome. Their study included the data obtained from 3719 patients with takotsubo syndrome between 2010 and 2013. Of these, 3300 patients were outpatients, and 419 were inpatients. The hospital mortality was significantly higher in the inpatients than outpatients (17.9% vs 5.4%; $P < .001$). The multivariable logistic regression analysis indicated that the hospital mortality of inpatients was twice than that of outpatients (odds ratio, 2.02; 95% CI, 1.43–2.85; $P < .001$).[36] As

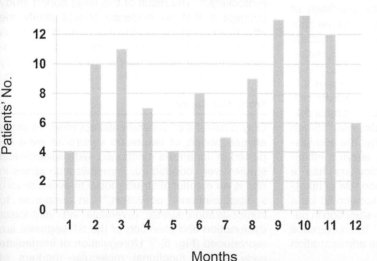

Fig. 4. Seasonal distribution of onset of takotsubo syndrome. The bimodal peaks in spring and autumn are suggested. (*Adapted from* Murakami T, Yoshikawa T, Maekawa Y, et al. Characterization of predictors of in-hospital cardiac complications of takotsubo cardiomyopathy: multi-center registry from Tokyo CCU Network. J Cardiol 2014;63:270; with permission.)

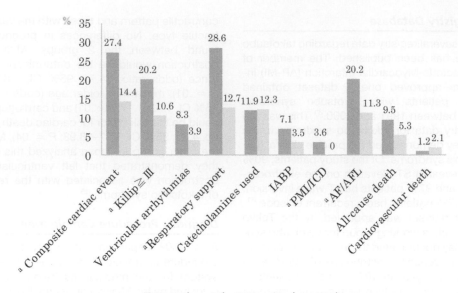

■ Male (n = 84)   ■ Female (n = 284)

Fig. 5. Composite cardiac events are defined as cardiovascular death, severe pump failure, or serious ventricular arrhythmias, such as ventricular tachycardia/ventricular fibrillation (VT/VF). AF/AFL, atrial fibrillation or flutter; IABP, intraaortic balloon pump; Killip, Killip class; PMI/ICD, implantation of pacemaker or cardioverter-defibrillator; VT/VF, ventricular arrhythmias; respiratory support, mechanical ventilation or noninvasive positive pressure ventilation. [a] P < .05. (*Adapted from* Murakami T, Yoshikawa T, Maekawa Y, et al. Gender differences in patients with takotsubo cardiomyopathy: multi-center registry from Tokyo CCU Network. PLoS One 2015;10:e0136655; with permission.)

previously reported outside Japan, the mortality after discharge is remarkably unfavorable and it depends on the first 4 years after diagnosis. The prognosis is determined by the presence or absence of noncardiac illness,[37] even in the short-term prognosis.[36]

Treatment

No randomized trials have demonstrated the effectiveness of preventing lethal complications or treatment for wall motion abnormalities. The mortality depends on the baseline condition of the patients; secondary takotsubo syndrome after a critical disease was much worse. The in-hospital mortalities of takotsubo patients are reported 6.8% from the large cohort study conducted in Japan[36] and 4.5% from the world metaanalysis.[38] The in-hospital mortality of Japanese patients with takotsubo syndrome, 6.8%, is lethal comparable with that of patients with AMI in this era.[39] Singh and colleagues[40] have reported that the administration of angiotensin-converting enzyme inhibitors or angiotensin receptor blockers has a potential to decrease the recurrence rate of takotsubo syndrome. Although β-blockers could be a protective option for myocardial dysfunction in patients with takotsubo syndrome,[41] the recurrence is reported under the usual dosage administration with β-blockers.[40,42]

Isogai and colleagues[43] recently analyzed the nationwide data based on the diagnosis procedure combination database and presented the mortality of patients with takotsubo syndrome under early β-blocker administration in Japan. Of the 2672 patients, 423 received β-blockers within 2 days after the onset (early β-blocker group) and the remaining patients received β-blockers 3 days or more thereafter (control group). They demonstrated neither a beneficial nor harmful result regardless of the initiation time of β-blockers.[43] The result of this large cohort study suggested that no evidence should clarify the effectiveness of early β-blocker administration as a routine option for patients with takotsubo syndrome in their acute phase. This result is only limited in Japanese patients, not in global patients.

From the Bench

Only a handful of experimental approaches using animal models of takotsubo syndrome were reported in Japan. As mentioned, extensive clinical studies were conducted. Immobilization stress in rats is an emotional stress model to evoke severe sympathoadrenal activation.[44] In response to immobilization stress, reversible left ventricular dysfunction and elevation of the ST-segment are reproduced (**Fig. 6**).[45] Upregulation of immediate early genes, functional molecular markers of

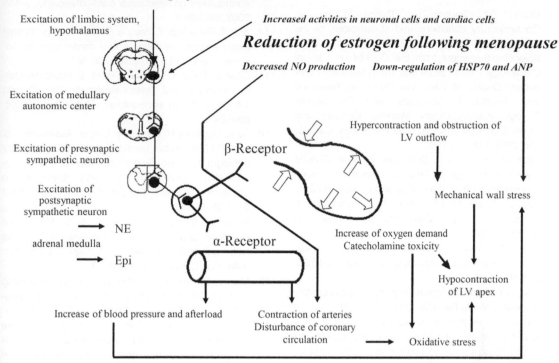

Fig. 6. Possible underlying mechanism of typical takotsubo syndrome. ANP, atrial natriuretic peptide; Epi, epinephrine; LV, left ventricular; NE, norepinephrine; NO, nitric oxide. (*Adapted from* Akashi YJ, Goldstein DS, Barbaro G, et al. Takotsubo cardiomyopathy: a new form of acute, reversible heart failure. Circulation 2008;118:2754–62; with permission.)

cellular activation, and transcriptional factors are observed in the myocardium and the coronary arteries. These physiologic and molecular alterations are completely prevented by pretreatment with αβ-blockers, suggesting that pathologic increased sympathoadrenal activity should underlie the etiology of stress cardiomyopathy. The effect of αβ-adrenoceptor blockers on the prevention of stress-induced cardiac dysfunction has been recently confirmed.[46] A calcium channel blocker, azelnidipine, prevents a decrease of cardiac systolic function in a rat model.[47] Acute premedication with β-blockers also prevent cardiac dysfunction in a rat model,[48] although the negative results using β-blockers in patients with takotsubo syndrome have been reported. The same researchers suggested that oxidative stress response should be the underlying mechanism.

There is a trend toward an higher prevalence of takotsubo syndrome in postmenopausal women whose estrogen concentrations are diminished. Treatment with estrogen attenuates stress-induced neuronal excitation in the central sympathetic neurons and neurons with immunoreactive estrogen receptors.[49] It also decreases the activation of the adrenal gland and the heart; that is,

estrogen attenuates the stress-induced hypothalamosympathoadrenal outflow from the central nervous system to the target organs. Estrogen treatment also upregulates the levels of cardioprotective substances in the heart.[49] Because this treatment method is still a future option for takotsubo syndrome, further research is called for.

SUMMARY

This paper summarizes the evidence originally presented from Japan. Takotsubo syndrome is a newly described heart failure characterized by transient left ventricular dysfunction. Although the pathogenesis of this syndrome remains unclear, Japanese researchers conducted various studies to investigate the profound mechanisms from bench to bedside. We should be aware of this entity as a syndrome, not actual cardiomyopathy. Japanese researchers focus on the experimental approaches for clinical diagnosis and treatment of takotsubo syndrome. As representatives from a country originally naming this syndrome takotsubo, a global registry for takotsubo syndrome including Japan should be established.

REFERENCES

1. Maron BJ, Towbin JA, Thiene G, et al. Contemporary definitions and classification of the cardiomyopathies: an American Heart Association Scientific Statement from the Council on Clinical Cardiology, Heart Failure and Transplantation Committee; Quality of Care and Outcomes Research and Functional Genomics and Translational Biology Interdisciplinary Working Groups; and Council on Epidemiology and Prevention. Circulation 2006;113:1807–16.

2. Lyon AR, Bossone E, Schneider B, et al. Current state of knowledge on Takotsubo syndrome: a position statement from the taskforce on Takotsubo Syndrome of the Heart Failure Association of the European Society of Cardiology. Eur J Heart Fail 2016;18:8–27.

3. Akashi YJ, Takano M, Miyake F. Scintigraphic imaging in Tako-Tsubo cardiomyopathy. Herz 2010;35:231–9.

4. Akashi YJ, Nef HM, Mollmann H, et al. Stress cardiomyopathy. Annu Rev Med 2010;61:271–86.

5. Yoshioka T, Hashimoto A, Tsuchihashi K, et al. Clinical implications of midventricular obstruction and intravenous propranolol use in transient left ventricular apical ballooning (Tako-tsubo cardiomyopathy). Am Heart J 2008;155(526):e1–7.

6. Peters MN, George P, Irimpen AM. The broken heart syndrome: Takotsubo cardiomyopathy. Trends Cardiovasc Med 2015;25:351–7.

7. Sato H, Tateishi H, Dote K, et al. Tako-tsubo-like left ventricular dysfunction due to multivessel coronary spasm. In: Kodama K, Haze K, Hon M, editors. Clinical aspect of myocardial injury: from ischemia to heart failure. Tokyo: Kagakuhyouronsha; 1990. p. 56–64.

8. Dote K, Sato H, Tateishi H, et al. Myocardial stunning due to simultaneous multivessel coronary spasms: a review of 5 cases. J Cardiol 1991;21:203–14 [in Japanese].

9. Case records of the Massachusetts General Hospital. Weekly clinicopathological exercises. Case 18-1986. A 44-year-old woman with substernal pain and pulmonary edema after severe emotional stress. N Engl J Med 1986;314:1240–7.

10. Kuramoto K, Matsushita S, Murakami M. Acute reversible myocardial infarction after blood transfusion in the aged. Jpn Heart J 1977;18:191–201.

11. Yamabe H, Hanaoka J, Funakoshi T, et al. Deep negative T waves and abnormal cardiac sympathetic image (123I-MIBG) after the Great Hanshin Earthquake of 1995. Am J Med Sci 1996;311:221–4.

12. Ogawa K, Tsuji I, Shiono K, et al. Increased acute myocardial infarction mortality following the 1995 Great Hanshin-Awaji earthquake in Japan. Int J Epidemiol 2000;29:449–55.

13. Watanabe H, Kodama M, Okura Y, et al. Impact of earthquakes on Takotsubo cardiomyopathy. JAMA 2005;294:305–7.

14. Aoki T, Fukumoto Y, Yasuda S, et al. The great east japan earthquake disaster and cardiovascular diseases. Eur Heart J 2012;33:2796–803.

15. Chan C, Elliott J, Troughton R, et al. Acute myocardial infarction and stress cardiomyopathy following the Christchurch earthquakes. PLoS One 2013;8:e68504.

16. Ito K, Sugihara H, Kawasaki T, et al. Assessment of ampulla (Takotsubo) cardiomyopathy with coronary angiography, two-dimensional echocardiography and 99mTc-tetrofosmin myocardial single photon emission computed tomography. Ann Nucl Med 2001;15:351–5.

17. Kurisu S, Inoue I, Kawagoe T, et al. Myocardial perfusion and fatty acid metabolism in patients with tako-tsubo-like left ventricular dysfunction. J Am Coll Cardiol 2003;41:743–8.

18. Matsuo S, Nakajima K, Kinuya S, et al. Diagnostic utility of 123I-BMIPP imaging in patients with Takotsubo cardiomyopathy. J Cardiol 2014;64:49–56.

19. Owa M, Aizawa K, Urasawa N, et al. Emotional stress-induced 'ampulla cardiomyopathy' discrepancy between the metabolic and sympathetic innervation imaging performed during the recovery course. Jpn Circ J 2001;65:349–52.

20. Ito K, Sugihara H, Kinoshita N, et al. Assessment of Takotsubo cardiomyopathy (transient left ventricular apical ballooning) using 99mTc-tetrofosmin, 123I-BMIPP, 123I-MIBG and 99mTc-PYP myocardial SPECT. Ann Nucl Med 2005;19:435–45.

21. Akashi YJ, Nakazawa K, Sakakibara M, et al. 123I-MIBG myocardial scintigraphy in patients with "takotsubo" cardiomyopathy. J Nucl Med 2004;45:1121–7.

22. Humbert O, Stamboul K, Gudjoncik A, et al. Dual diagnostic role of 123I-MIBG scintigraphy in inverted-takotsubo pattern cardiomyopathy. Clin Nucl Med 2015;40:816–8.

23. Akashi YJ, Barbaro G, Sakurai T, et al. Cardiac autonomic imbalance in patients with reversible ventricular dysfunction takotsubo cardiomyopathy. Q J Med 2007;100:335–43.

24. Yoshida T, Hibino T, Kako N, et al. A pathophysiologic study of tako-tsubo cardiomyopathy with F-18 fluorodeoxyglucose positron emission tomography. Eur Heart J 2007;28:2598–604.

25. Miyachi H, Kumita S, Tanaka K. PET/CT and SPECT/CT cardiac fusion imaging in a patient with takotsubo cardiomyopathy. Eur Heart J 2013;34:397.

26. Izumo M, Nalawadi S, Shiota M, et al. Mechanisms of acute mitral regurgitation in patients with takotsubo cardiomyopathy: an echocardiographic study. Circ Cardiovasc Imaging 2011;4:392–8.

27. Izumo M, Shiota M, Nalawadi S, et al. Determinants of secondary pulmonary hypertension in patients with takotsubo cardiomyopathy. Echocardiography 2015;32:1608–13.

28. Kosuge M, Ebina T, Hibi K, et al. Simple and accurate electrocardiographic criteria to differentiate takotsubo cardiomyopathy from anterior acute myocardial infarction. J Am Coll Cardiol 2010;55:2514–6.

29. Kosuge M, Ebina T, Hibi K, et al. Differences in negative T waves among acute coronary syndrome, acute pulmonary embolism, and Takotsubo cardiomyopathy. Eur Heart J Acute Cardiovasc Care 2012;1:349–57.

30. Shimizu M, Nishizaki M, Yamawake N, et al. J wave and fragmented QRS formation during the hyperacute phase in Takotsubo cardiomyopathy. Circ J 2014;78:943–9.

31. Tsuchihashi K, Ueshima K, Uchida T, et al. Transient left ventricular apical ballooning without coronary artery stenosis: a novel heart syndrome mimicking acute myocardial infarction. Angina pectoris-myocardial infarction investigations in Japan. J Am Coll Cardiol 2001;38:11–8.

32. Murakami T, Yoshikawa T, Maekawa Y, et al. Characterization of predictors of in-hospital cardiac complications of takotsubo cardiomyopathy: multi-center registry from Tokyo CCU Network. J Cardiol 2014;63:269–73.

33. Murakami T, Yoshikawa T, Maekawa Y, et al. Gender differences in patients with Takotsubo cardiomyopathy: multi-center registry from Tokyo CCU Network. PLoS One 2015;10:e0136655.

34. Nishida J, Kouzu H, Hashimoto A, et al. "Ballooning" patterns in takotsubo cardiomyopathy reflect different clinical backgrounds and outcomes: a BOREAS-TCM study. Heart Vessels 2015;30:789–97.

35. Kawaji T, Shiomi H, Morimoto T, et al. Clinical impact of left ventricular outflow tract obstruction in takotsubo cardiomyopathy. Circ J 2015;79:839–46.

36. Isogai T, Yasunaga H, Matsui H, et al. Out-of-hospital versus in-hospital Takotsubo cardiomyopathy: analysis of 3719 patients in the diagnosis procedure combination database in Japan. Int J Cardiol 2014;176:413–7.

37. Song BG, Hahn JY, Cho SJ, et al. Clinical characteristics, ballooning pattern, and long-term prognosis of transient left ventricular ballooning syndrome. Heart Lung 2010;39:188–95.

38. Singh K, Carson K, Shah R, et al. Meta-analysis of clinical correlates of acute mortality in takotsubo cardiomyopathy. Am J Cardiol 2014;113:1420–8.

39. Ishihara M, Fujino M, Ogawa H, et al. Clinical presentation, management and outcome of Japanese patients with acute myocardial infarction in the troponin era - Japanese Registry of Acute Myocardial Infarction Diagnosed by Universal Definition (J-MINUET). Circ J 2015;79:1255–62.

40. Singh K, Carson K, Usmani Z, et al. Systematic review and meta-analysis of incidence and correlates of recurrence of takotsubo cardiomyopathy. Int J Cardiol 2014;174:696–701.

41. Akashi YJ, Nef HM, Lyon AR. Epidemiology and pathophysiology of Takotsubo syndrome. Nat Rev Cardiol 2015;12:387–97.

42. Santoro F, Ieva R, Musaico F, et al. Lack of efficacy of drug therapy in preventing takotsubo cardiomyopathy recurrence: a meta-analysis. Clin Cardiol 2014;37:434–9.

43. Isogai T, Matsui H, Tanaka H, et al. Early beta-blocker use and in-hospital mortality in patients with Takotsubo cardiomyopathy. Heart 2016;102(13):1029–35.

44. Kvetnansky R, Weise VK, Thoa NB, et al. Effects of chronic guanethidine treatment and adrenal medullectomy on plasma levels of catecholamines and corticosterone in forcibly immobilized rats. J Pharmacol Exp Ther 1979;209:287–91.

45. Akashi YJ, Goldstein DS, Barbaro G, et al. Takotsubo cardiomyopathy: a new form of acute, reversible heart failure. Circulation 2008;118:2754–62.

46. Uchida M, Egawa M, Yamaguchi S, et al. Protective effects of emotional stress-induced cardiac dysfunction depend on α/β ratio of adrenoceptor blocker. Circ J 2009;73(Suppl 1):595.

47. Takano Y, Ueyama T, Ishikura F. Azelnidipine, unique calcium channel blocker could prevent stress-induced cardiac dysfunction like alpha.beta blocker. J Cardiol 2012;60:18–22.

48. Ishikura F, Takano Y, Ueyama T. Acute effects of beta-blocker with intrinsic sympathomimetic activity on stress-induced cardiac dysfunction in rats. J Cardiol 2012;60(6):470–4.

49. Ueyama T, Kasamatsu K, Hano T, et al. Catecholamines and estrogen are involved in the pathogenesis of emotional stress-induced acute heart attack. Ann N Y Acad Sci 2008;1148:479–85.

The International Takotsubo Registry
Rationale, Design, Objectives, and First Results

Jelena-R. Ghadri, MD*, Victoria L. Cammann,
Christian Templin, MD, PhD

KEYWORDS

- Takotsubo syndrome • Broken heart syndrome • Cardiomyopathy • Heart failure
- International Takotsubo Registry

KEY POINTS

- Takotsubo syndrome (TTS) was first described in the early 1990s and is still poorly understood; the underlying disease mechanism is unknown.
- Knowledge on TTS is mainly derived from case reports, series, or small-scale single-center studies. To overcome the challenge of small patient numbers, a registry approach is required.
- The International Takotsubo Registry (InterTAK Registry) aims to advance the understanding of TTS and to improve diagnosis, treatment, and outcomes of this puzzling disease.

INTRODUCTION

Takotsubo syndrome (TTS) is characterized by the acute onset of left ventricular dysfunction with specific wall motion patterns usually precipitated by physical or emotional stress.[1,2] Interestingly, TTS predominantly affects postmenopausal women.[2–4] Sign and symptom complex is similar to that of acute coronary syndrome (ACS); therefore, TTS should be considered in the differential diagnosis for acute chest pain.[5] It is likely that many TTS cases remain unreported because of being misdiagnosed as ACS.[5,6] Although several acute complications such as heart failure, arrhythmias, cardiogenic shock, and even death can occur,[2,5] TTS is commonly believed to be a benign disorder. However, outcome studies are scarce and mainly based on small patient numbers.[3,7] Furthermore, there is no international and unifying definition for TTS because its clinical features have not been elucidated fully. In addition, there are no established guidelines for therapeutic management of TTS because randomized trials are currently lacking.[5]

To address incomplete knowledge on TTS and low prevalence of reported cases a registry approach was implemented by establishing the

Disclosure Statement: C. Templin reports receiving fees for serving on advisory boards from Abbott Vascular and Boston Scientific; fees for training in transcatheter aortic-valve implantation from Boston Scientific, Edwards Lifesciences, and Medtronic; travel support from Abbott Vascular, Boston Scientific, Biosensors, Edwards Lifesciences, and Medtronic; and grant support from Abbott Vascular and Biosensors.
Funding: J.-R. Ghadri was supported by "Filling the gap", a research grant from the University of Zurich, V.L. Cammann was supported by a research grant from the Foundation of Cardiovascular Research, Zurich Heart House.
Department of Cardiology, University Heart Center, University Hospital Zurich, Raemistrasse 100, Zurich 8091, Switzerland
* Corresponding author.
E-mail address: Jelena-Rima.Ghadri@usz.ch

Heart Failure Clin 12 (2016) 597–603
http://dx.doi.org/10.1016/j.hfc.2016.06.010
1551-7136/16/$ – see front matter © 2016 Elsevier Inc. All rights reserved.

International Takotsubo Registry (InterTAK Registry; www.takotsubo-registry.com), a multinational collaborative network. Currently more than 35 international cardiovascular centers from 15 countries are collaborating in this unique registry, including centers in Argentina, Australia, Austria, the Czech Republic, Denmark, Finland, France, Germany, Italy, New Zealand, Poland, Portugal, Switzerland, the United Kingdom, and the United States (**Fig. 1**).

RATIONALE BEHIND THE INTERNATIONAL TAKOTSUBO REGISTRY

Despite numerous publications on TTS, a major problem of virtually all studies of TTS is the relatively small patient number, mainly owing to the low disease prevalence. In addition, incomplete knowledge of its clinical features, management, and outcomes prompted us to create a powerful and comprehensive knowledge base using a registry approach to study unanswered questions, increase the reliability of data, and advance the understanding of this complex disease. Collecting clinical information through a registry can be extremely valuable in studying particularly a "rare

disease."[8,9] As such, data can be obtained from a large, more heterogeneous and geographically diverse patient population than those collected from a single-center study and the results provide a more valid basis for generalization.

DESIGN OF THE INTERNATIONAL TAKOTSUBO REGISTRY

The InterTAK Registry is designed as an international, multicenter, prospective and retrospective, observational study of patients with TTS (ClinicalTrials.gov identifier: NCT01947621). Male and female patients with the diagnosis of TTS are included in the InterTAK Registry; all patients with myocarditis are excluded. The diagnosis of TTS is based on modified Mayo Clinic Diagnostic Criteria, including[2,10] (i) transient left ventricular hypokinesia, akinesia, or dyskinesia that extends beyond a single coronary artery perfusion territory (exceptions are the focal TTS type in whom the regional wall motion abnormality is limited to a single epicardial coronary distribution), (ii) absence of obstructive coronary artery disease or angiographic evidence of acute plaque rupture (note: it is possible that a patient with obstructive coronary

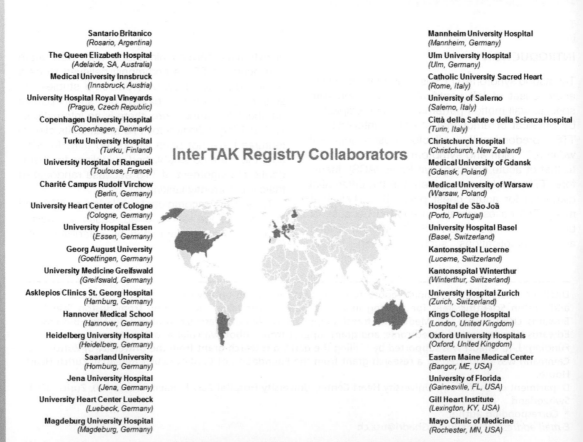

Santario Britanico
(Rosario, Argentina)

The Queen Elizabeth Hospital
(Adelaide, SA, Australia)

Medical University Innsbruck
(Innsbruck, Austria)

University Hospital Royal Vineyards
(Prague, Czech Republic)

Copenhagen University Hospital
(Copenhagen, Denmark)

Turku University Hospital
(Turku, Finland)

University Hospital of Rangueil
(Toulouse, France)

Charité Campus Rudolf Virchow
(Berlin, Germany)

University Heart Center of Cologne
(Cologne, Germany)

University Hospital Essen
(Essen, Germany)

Georg August University
(Goettingen, Germany)

University Medicine Greifswald
(Greifswald, Germany)

Asklepios Clinics St. Georg Hospital
(Hamburg, Germany)

Hannover Medical School
(Hannover, Germany)

Heidelberg University Hospital
(Heidelberg, Germany)

Saarland University
(Homburg, Germany)

Jena University Hospital
(Jena, Germany)

University Heart Center Luebeck
(Luebeck, Germany)

Magdeburg University Hospital
(Magdeburg, Germany)

InterTAK Registry Collaborators

Mannheim University Hospital
(Mannheim, Germany)

Ulm University Hospital
(Ulm, Germany)

Catholic University Sacred Heart
(Rome, Italy)

University of Salerno
(Salerno, Italy)

Città della Salute e della Scienza Hospital
(Turin, Italy)

Christchurch Hospital
(Christchurch, New Zealand)

Medical University of Gdansk
(Gdansk, Poland)

Medical University of Warsaw
(Warsaw, Poland)

Hospital de São Joã
(Porto, Portugal)

University Hospital Basel
(Basel, Switzerland)

Kantonsspital Lucerne
(Lucerne, Switzerland)

Kantonsspital Winterthur
(Winterthur, Switzerland)

University Hospital Zurich
(Zurich, Switzerland)

Kings College Hospital
(London, United Kingdom)

Oxford University Hospitals
(Oxford, United Kingdom)

Eastern Maine Medical Center
(Bangor, ME, USA)

University of Florida
(Gainesville, FL, USA)

Gill Heart Institute
(Lexington, KY, USA)

Mayo Clinic of Medicine
(Rochester, MN, USA)

Fig. 1. Collaborating centers of the International Takotsubo Registry (InterTAK Registry).

atherosclerosis may also develop TTS), and (iii) new electrocardiographic (ECG) abnormalities (i.e., either ST-segment elevation and/or T-wave inversion) or a modest elevation in cardiac troponin levels. When eligibility for inclusion in the registry remains uncertain, all members of the core team examine the case to reach agreement.[2]

Demographic characteristics, laboratory values, ECG parameters, coronary angiography and echocardiographic findings, triggering factors (categorized as emotional and/or physical), cardiovascular risk factors, coexisting illnesses, use of medications, critical care, and outcomes are collected systematically for all patients with standardized forms to obtain as much information as possible. Based on the region of the wall motion abnormality different TTS types are classified as apical (defined as typical), midventricular, basal, or focal (all defined as atypical) forms.[2,11]

In addition to the registry, we have integrated a biobank, which is an excellent tool to study genetic factors and biomarkers of TTS.[12]

OBJECTIVES OF THE INTERNATIONAL TAKOTSUBO REGISTRY

The InterTAK Registry aims to provide a unique, worldwide database on a large number of patients to shed light on this multifaceted clinical entity. The goals of the InterTAK Registry are to determine the disease epidemiology, clinical features, and outcomes as well as to improve treatment strategies. Furthermore, it is designed to investigate the patho-physiologic mechanisms, identify diagnostic and prognostic factors in terms of biomarkers, and explore the genetic basis of the disease (**Fig. 2**). Another scope is to enhance education not only among health professionals but also among patients. Data of the InterTAK Registry will expand the knowledge and generate novel insights into this fascinating disease ultimately leading to an improved patient care. Finally, the registry results may have the potential to represent an important cornerstone for future prospective trials.

FIRST RESULTS OF THE INTERNATIONAL TAKOTSUBO REGISTRY
Novel Clinical Features

First results of the InterTAK Registry representing the largest series of patients with this disorder show novel insights into clinical features, outcomes, and treatment. Furthermore, potential diagnostic biomarkers have been established and possible disease-related factors identified.

Our first results of the registry indicate that the majority of the 1750 analyzed patients are female

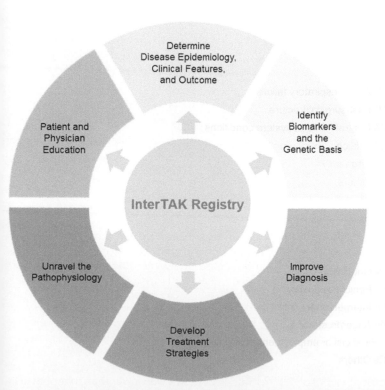

Fig. 2. Objectives of the International Takotsubo Registry (InterTAK Registry).

(female-to-male ratio, 9:1) and interestingly more prone to emotional stressors.[2] A unique feature of TTS is a preceding stressful event triggering the disease. In our study cohort, only 71.5% had a definite preceding trigger. Specifically, about one-quarter of patients had an emotional trigger, slightly more than one-third experienced a physical triggering event, and the remainder had no evident (28.5%) or a combination of physical and emotional (7.8%) stressors (**Fig. 3**).[2] Contrary to previously published studies,[3,4] we found that in the overall population, men presenting with TTS were on average significantly younger than women (62.9 ± 13.1 vs 66.8 ± 13.0 years).[2] Furthermore, it has been revealed that TTS is more heterogeneous and affects a wider range of patients than previously assumed.[2] Younger patients, men, those without an emotional trigger, and individuals who present with other severe illness such as an acute cerebral hemorrhage or an acute psychiatric episode can all develop TTS. Notably, we have demonstrated that patients with TTS had a higher prevalence of neurologic and psychiatric disorders than those with ACS.[2] Therefore, it is conceivable that there is a causal relationship between neurologic and psychiatric diseases and the susceptibility to develop TTS in terms of an activated brain–heart interaction.

In contrast with the common belief that patients with TTS have no coronary artery stenosis, we found that 15.3% of patients with TTS had also evidence of concomitant coronary artery disease.[2] Thus, the coexistence of coronary artery disease does not exclude the diagnosis of TTS.

Since the first description of TTS, small-scale clinical studies have shown that variants exist.[13,14] Besides the distinctive apical ballooning,[1] midventricular,[15] basal,[16] or focal[17]

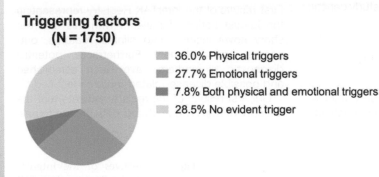

Triggering factors (N = 1750)

- 36.0% Physical triggers
- 27.7% Emotional triggers
- 7.8% Both physical and emotional triggers
- 28.5% No evident trigger

Fig. 3. Triggering factors in takotsubo syndrome. (*From* Templin C, Ghadri JR, Diekmann J, et al. Clinical features and outcomes of takotsubo (stress) cardiomyopathy. N Engl J Med 2015;373:929–38; with permission.)

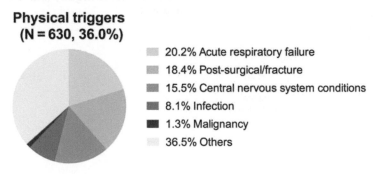

Physical triggers (N = 630, 36.0%)

- 20.2% Acute respiratory failure
- 18.4% Post-surgical/fracture
- 15.5% Central nervous system conditions
- 8.1% Infection
- 1.3% Malignancy
- 36.5% Others

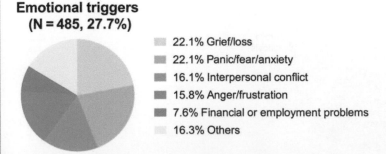

Emotional triggers (N = 485, 27.7%)

- 22.1% Grief/loss
- 22.1% Panic/fear/anxiety
- 16.1% Interpersonal conflict
- 15.8% Anger/frustration
- 7.6% Financial or employment problems
- 16.3% Others

wall motion abnormalities of the left ventricle have been noted, although the source of the differences remains unknown. Because data from patients with atypical forms of TTS are limited, clinical features of these subgroups are not well-described.

We have shown recently that the typical apical ballooning occurs in about 80% of patients and atypical subtypes (i.e., midventricular, basal, and focal TTS type) represent the remaining 20% of cases (**Fig. 4**).[2,11] Notably, we identified more atypical cases during the later years of the study period suggesting that TTS variations are being recognized more frequently than they have been in the past.[11]

Atypical TTS has different clinical characteristics than typical TTS, including younger patient age, more frequent ST-segment depression, higher prevalence of neurologic disease, less impaired left ventricular ejection fraction, and lower brain natriuretic peptide values.[11] Patients with typical and atypical TTS reveal comparable in-hospital complication rates and outcomes.[11] A left ventricular ejection fraction of less than 45%, atrial

fibrillation, and the presence of neurologic disease, but not the TTS type emerged as independent predictors of death at 1-year follow-up.[11]

Based on our comprehensive database from the InterTAK Registry, we have identified for the first time by a large systematic collection of patients with a definite emotional trigger (n = 485) that also positive life events (n = 20) can trigger TTS by terming this condition "happy heart syndrome".[18] These positive life events included for instance jackpot win, birthday party, son's wedding, a positive job interview, or becoming grandmother. Although the clinical presentation and outcomes were comparable; in a post-hoc analysis patients with a happy heart syndrome demonstrated a higher prevalence of a midventricular ballooning pattern than patients with a negative emotional trigger (35.0% vs 16.3%; P = .030).[18] Because these results cannot be explained so far, this is an interesting observation that needs to be investigated further. These findings show that triggers for TTS can be more varied than previously thought and should lead to a paradigm shift in clinical practice.[18]

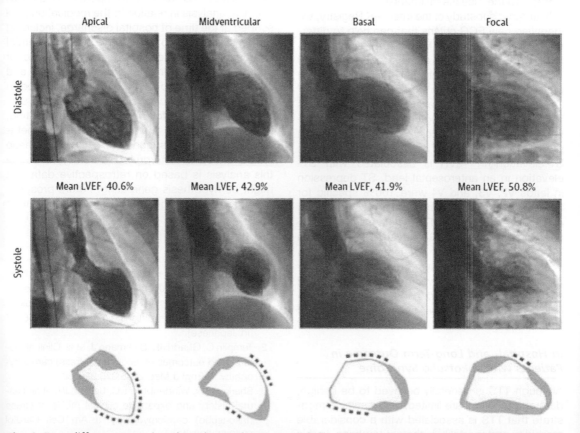

Fig. 4. Four different types in takotsubo syndrome. LVEF, left ventricular ejection fraction. (*From* Ghadri JR, Cammann VL, Napp LC, et al. Differences in the clinical profile and outcomes of typical and atypical takotsubo syndrome. Ghadri JR, Cammann VL, Napp LC, et al. JAMA Cardiol 2016;1(3):335–40; with permission.)

New Diagnostic Features Focusing on Biomarkers and Electrocardiography

In its early clinical presentation, TTS is indistinguishable from ACS. As such, in TTS levels of cardiac biomarkers including troponin and creatine kinase are increased. Therefore, there is an urgent need to identify specific markers that allow rapid noninvasive diagnosis in the acute phase of TTS. We have recently identified a signature of 4 circulating microRNAs (miR-16, miR-26a, miR-1, and miR-133a) with a good sensitivity and specificity that may serve as biomarkers to distinguish TTS from myocardial infarction (MI) in its early clinical presentation.[12]

The upregulation of the serum and depression related miR-16 and miR-26 suggests a strong link to neuropsychiatric disorders. A decrease of the endothelin-1 regulatory miRNA125a-5p was measured. Notably, we found a significant increase in endothelin-1, which implies that there is a potential role of endothelin-1 as a mediator of microvascular spasm.[12] Therefore, our results highlight that linking a registry to a biobank can enhance scientific research and give important insights into the disease mechanism.

In another substudy of the InterTAK Registry, we identified new ECG criteria that can help to differentiate TTS from acute MI on admission. Therefore, we compared the admission ECGs of 200 TTS patients from our InterTAK Registry with 200 patients of MI from the Zurich ACS Registry.[19] The comparison of ST-elevation MI (STEMI) versus TTS patients with ST-segment elevation demonstrated a 100% specificity and 100% positive predictive value for the diagnosis of TTS, when ST-elevation in –aVR is associated with ST-elevation in an anteroseptal lead. ST depression in leads V2, V3, and V4 were 100% specific for STEMI. Comparing patients with non–ST-segment elevation NSTEMI to TTS patients with non–ST-segment elevation, ST-elevation in –aVR with T-inversion in any other lead revealed a 100% specificity (100% positive predictive value) for the diagnosis of TTS, whereas the presence of ST depression in leads V2 and V3 were 99% specific for NSTEMI with a positive predictive value of 91% in the same setting.[19]

In-Hospital- and Long-Term Outcome in Patients with Takotsubo Syndrome

Although TTS is generally believed to be benign, data on outcomes are limited. Our results demonstrate that TTS is associated with a considerable morbidity and mortality in the acute phase. In this regard, 21.8% of TTS patients experienced the composite endpoint of serious in-hospital complications.[2] Particularly, rates of cardiogenic shock and in-hospital death were similar to the rates of an age- and sex-matched cohort of patients presenting with ACS, most of these endpoints, including in-hospital death, occurred more frequently in males than in females.[2]

Multivariate analysis revealed that older age and the presence of emotional triggers independently predicted a lower incidence of the composite endpoint.[2]

In contrast, the presence of physical triggers, acute neurologic or psychiatric disease, an admission troponin measurement of more than 10 times the upper limit of the normal range, and a left ventricular ejection fraction of less than 45% were associated with an unfavorable outcome for the composite endpoint.[2] Even after the acute phase, long-term outcome is not benign. The risk of major adverse cardiac and cerebrovascular events was 9.9% per patient-year and the risk for death 5.6% per patient-year.[2]

Outcome in Relation to Medication

No randomized trials or guidelines exist for the treatment of TTS. We therefore performed a retrospective analysis in relation to the medication prescribed at the time of hospital discharge, including propensity scores to reduce the bias to potential confounding variables. Interestingly, the use of angiotensin-converting enzyme inhibitors and angiotensin receptor blockers, but not beta-blockers, was associated with an improved survival after 1 year of follow-up.[2] This is interesting, because a possible therapeutic benefit of beta-blockers has been suggested.[20] However, these results must be interpreted carefully, because this analysis is based on retrospective data and might be hypothesis generating. Future prospective studies are needed to confirm these results.

REFERENCES

1. Sato H. Tako-tsubo-like left ventricular dysfunction due to multivessel coronary spasm. In: Kodama K, Haze K, Hori M, editors. Clinical aspect of myocardial injury: from Ischemia to heart failure. Tokyo: Kagakuhyoronsha Publishing Co; 1990. p. 56–64 [in Japanese].

2. Templin C, Ghadri JR, Diekmann J, et al. Clinical features and outcomes of takotsubo (stress) cardiomyopathy. N Engl J Med 2015;373:929–38.

3. Sharkey SW, Windenburg DC, Lesser JR, et al. Natural history and expansive clinical profile of stress (tako-tsubo) cardiomyopathy. J Am Coll Cardiol 2010;55:333–41.

4. Schneider B, Athanasiadis A, Stollberger C, et al. Gender differences in the manifestation of

tako-tsubo cardiomyopathy. Int J Cardiol 2013;166: 584–8.

5. Ghadri JR, Ruschitzka F, Luscher TF, et al. Takotsubo cardiomyopathy: still much more to learn. Heart 2014;100:1804–12.

6. Templin C, Napp LC, Ghadri JR. Takotsubo syndrome: underdiagnosed, underestimated, but understood? J Am Coll Cardiol 2016;67:1937–40.

7. Elesber AA, Prasad A, Lennon RJ, et al. Four-year recurrence rate and prognosis of the apical ballooning syndrome. J Am Coll Cardiol 2007;50: 448–52.

8. Moliner AM. Creating a European Union framework for actions in the field of rare diseases. Adv Exp Med Biol 2010;686:457–73.

9. Gliklich RE, Dreyer NA, Leavy MB, editors. Registries for evaluating patient outcomes: A user's guide. 3rd edition. Rockville (MD): Department of Health and Human Services USA; Agency for Healthcare Research and Quality; 2014.

10. Prasad A, Lerman A, Rihal CS. Apical ballooning syndrome (Tako-Tsubo or stress cardiomyopathy): a mimic of acute myocardial infarction. Am Heart J 2008;155:408–17.

11. Ghadri JR, Cammann VL, Napp LC, et al. Differences in the clinical profile and outcomes of typical and atypical takotsubo syndrome. JAMA Cardiol 2016;1(3):335–40.

12. Jaguszewski M, Osipova J, Ghadri JR, et al. A signature of circulating microRNAs differentiates takotsubo cardiomyopathy from acute myocardial infarction. Eur Heart J 2014;35:999–1006.

13. Shimizu M, Kato Y, Matsukawa R, et al. Recurrent severe mitral regurgitation due to left ventricular apical wall motion abnormality caused by coronary vasospastic angina: a case report. J Cardiol 2006; 47:31–7.

14. Nishida J, Kouzu H, Hashimoto A, et al. "Ballooning" patterns in takotsubo cardiomyopathy reflect different clinical backgrounds and outcomes: a BOREAS-TCM study. Heart Vessels 2015;30:789–97.

15. Shimizu M, Takahashi H, Fukatsu Y, et al. Reversible left ventricular dysfunction manifesting as hyperkinesis of the basal and the apical areas with akinesis of the mid portion: a case report. J Cardiol 2003;41: 285–90 [in Japanese].

16. Ennezat PV, Pesenti-Rossi D, Aubert JM, et al. Transient left ventricular basal dysfunction without coronary stenosis in acute cerebral disorders: a novel heart syndrome (inverted Takotsubo). Echocardiography 2005;22:599–602.

17. Suzuki K, Osada N, Akasi YJ, et al. An atypical case of "Takotsubo cardiomyopathy" during alcohol withdrawal: abnormality in the transient left ventricular wall motion and a remarkable elevation in the ST segment. Intern Med 2004;43:300–5.

18. Ghadri JR, Sarcon A, Diekmann J, et al. Happy heart syndrome: role of positive emotional stress in takotsubo syndrome. Eur Heart J 2016. [Epub ahead of print].

19. Frangieh AH, Obeid S, Ghadri JR, et al. ECG criteria to differentiate between takotsubo (stress) cardiomyopathy and infarction. J AM Hear Assoc 2016.

20. Kyuma M, Tsuchihashi K, Shinshi Y, et al. Effect of intravenous propranolol on left ventricular apical ballooning without coronary artery stenosis (ampulla cardiomyopathy): three cases. Circ J 2002;66:1181–4.

Moving?

Make sure your subscription moves with you!

To notify us of your new address, find your **Clinics Account Number** (located on your mailing label above your name), and contact customer service at:

Email: journalscustomerservice-usa@elsevier.com

800-654-2452 (subscribers in the U.S. & Canada)
314-447-8871 (subscribers outside of the U.S. & Canada)

Fax number: 314-447-8029

Elsevier Health Sciences Division
Subscription Customer Service
3251 Riverport Lane
Maryland Heights, MO 63043

*To ensure uninterrupted delivery of your subscription, please notify us at least 4 weeks in advance of move.

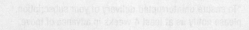

Printed and bound by CPI Group (UK) Ltd, Croydon, CR0 4YY

03/10/2024

01040298-0004